The Power
of the Voice

The Power
of the Voice

Lisbeth Hultmann
translated by Aileen Itani

AYNI
BOOKS

Winchester, UK
Washington, USA

First published by Ayni Books, 2013

Ayni Books is an imprint of John Hunt Publishing Ltd., Laurel House, Station Approach,
Alresford, Hants, SO24 9JH, UK
office1@jhpbooks.net
www.johnhuntpublishing.com
www.ayni-books.com

For distributor details and how to order please visit the 'Ordering' section on our website.

ISBN: 978 1 78099 938 8

A CIP catalogue record for this book is available from the British Library.

Design: Stuart Davies

Printed and bound by CPI Group (UK) Ltd, Croydon, CR0 4YY

We operate a distinctive and ethical publishing philosophy in all
areas of our business, from our global network of authors to
production and worldwide distribution.

Contents

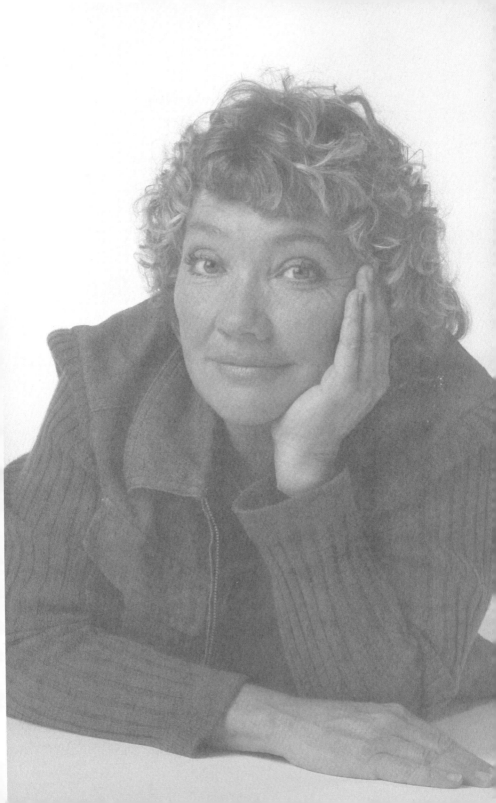

Foreword

Do you know what it's like, when you hear a voice that suddenly and without warning betrays a trembling insecurity behind the self-assured mask, becoming raspy and hoarse, cracked, or blocked by a lump in the throat?

Do you know what it's like, when a good friend only has to say "hi" on the phone, and you know immediately that something's wrong? Do you know those who—in certain situations—have to clear their throats constantly? Do you know the feeling of being manipulated, the feeling that you're picking up two sets of signals, when the words say one thing and the voice says something else? And do you know what it's like when two people can say the same thing and get totally different results, because you were certain one of them meant it, and the other didn't?

Have you met people who you associate with a particular character trait, because their voices seemed deadly monotone, absurdly girlish, erotic and tempting, or just bizarre, nasal and strained?

The voice reveals the body's secrets—but it is also a tool with which we can resolve our obstacles. Everything we forget, our body remembers. And everything the body remembers is reflected in the voice. With the help of vocal exercises we can work our way free of physical obstacles. And we can, on an unconscious level, wrench ourselves free of the traumas our obstacles conceal.

The voice is also a powerful tool for those who understand how to use it deliberately. It can close down all conversation or open up a long debate. We ask for abuse—and we give abuse—with our intonation and our phrasing; and the words we say can be less important than how we say them. The voice closes the deal—or bungles it for us—often leaving us totally unaware of why people do not respect us, why they fear us, or why they believe we are wonderful or insignificant.

Our conscious mind reacts to words, but our emotions react to the voice. Words can lie, but the voice never lies. Before one who understands how to interpret our voices, we are completely naked. And before one who understands how to use her voice deliberately, we are powerless—if we know nothing about how it works.

There is little in communication that we react to as strongly as voices. At the same time, there is little we are so oblivious to generally. Body language, how we dress—these have been discussed ad infinitum. Lisbeth Hultmann reveals the potential of the voice and its exciting, hidden universe.

Nanet Poulsen, journalist

Introduction

A word about me

I grew up with a spiritual background, because my parents were very interested in and inspired by the Danish thinker and philosopher Martinus. He left behind important writings about life's spiritual dimension. Even though I don't remember many details from my early childhood, I know that I learned early on that there is a deep meaning to everything. I think that it is this approach to life that has given me my basic optimism.

I have always considered my voice one of my greatest gifts. I began my singing career very early; my mother tells people I could sing before I could talk. As a two-year-old I could sit in a train or bus and hum without words. A lady once gave me two Danish crowns because she thought I sang so sweetly. The voice was my number one means of expression.

Later my path continued through the professional music world, where I acquired my stage and technical skills. As a child I sang in the Danish National Girls' Choir, and later with the Danish National Opera and in the Danish National Concert Choir. I felt, however, a growing desire to experiment more. I eventually broke on several occasions with the established music world in order to find my own way. The voice became the key to understanding myself, but not by using it in the traditional way. I had to free myself from the inflexible classical form in order to try new—and for me, more authentic and unorthodox—paths. For example, I worked for many years with modern dance and became certified as a movement teacher. Little by little I created my own combination of sound and movement. This combination became more intuitive: freer, and created in the moment. I have also, through multi-year therapeutic training, indulged my professional and personal curiosity, acquiring knowledge about the human psyche.

My path is stubbornly experimental, and I remain very

curious. I can now both give classical concerts without feeling bound by the style, and embrace other cultures' ways of using the voice, for example through intuitive singing. I stubbornly desire to be in contact with my inner self, and to stay open and sensitive to life and to my creative work. I see it as a necessary freedom, which not only I need, but we all need, in order to grow.

Origins of this book

This book has been a long time in coming. It started many years ago, when I felt I was working in a niche that had not been written about previously. It was like an uncultivated landscape, where I had to nourish the soil, plant and harvest all on my own. When I looked for literature on the voice, what I found discussed either speaking and singing technique, or more generally music and sound used as tools for personal growth, in which the voice played a vanishingly small part. A book that described the direct connection between voice and personality was not to be found. I was visited many times by people wanting to know more about the voice, who had themselves combed the literature looking for answers. This is my basis for thinking that there is a great interest in working with one's own voice in a context of personal growth, and a great need for knowledge about how the voice can be used.

In the beginning, I naïvely imagined that I would have to write a magnum opus, preferably in several volumes, and obviously only for specialists. Luckily I smartened up. First, when I was interviewed about the voice for a women's magazine, I became convinced that I should write my book immediately, and that it should be simple and brief. Two days after having this thought, a publisher contacted me and asked, "What about writing a book about the power of the voice?" From this my book got its name, which seemed self-evident to me; and it was hugely vindicating that someone else had had the same thought at the same time.

For this reason it has been a joy and a challenge to write this book. It is my hope that in the future there will be more research into the voice and its connection to the mind, and that more books will be written on the subject. For my own part, this will probably not be the last.

Who is this book for?

This book is for everyone who desires insight into the universe of the voice. It is about how we can change ourselves and the world around us by becoming more aware of the power of the voice. I hope that the book will bring joy and inspiration to all who desire change and growth. It is not a substitute for proper therapeutic work, but it can offer insight into how we can use the voice as a tool for our own development. It suggests simple tools for beginning your own process. I would suggest that you read the book a little at a time, rather than all at once. It is a good idea to get a feel for each chapter before reading further. Perhaps discuss it with others as well.

I do not recommend that persons with serious mental or vocal problems undertake the exercises in this book. The voice encompasses many resources capable of unleashing strong emotions that can be difficult to manage alone. In this case I would recommend for example that you go through the book with a professional therapist.

You can get just as much out of this book whether you are a professional singer or someone who has never trained his or her voice before. The book is about the voice as a part of human personality, but in the context of consciousness rather than technique. The voice is presented in a broader and more general perspective. Therefore your background and professional expertise are not essential, nor are they a prerequisite for deriving benefits from the book. It is my intention to reveal a more exalted perspective on the human voice—one from which every single person derives his or her unique and noble birthright.

Acknowledgements

I would first and foremost like to thank all the people who crossed my path in my teaching, and who thereby helped me gather experiences, for making this book possible. Next I would like to thank Nanet Poulsen, who helped me with the book, for her commitment and very positive support and encouragement. A warm thanks to Marianne Lykke for bringing clear-sightedness to her reading of the manuscript. Thanks to everyone who helped with the computer, and to all those who lovingly followed the process. A special thanks to my family, who from time to time were obliged to be very patient.

Lisbeth Hultmann

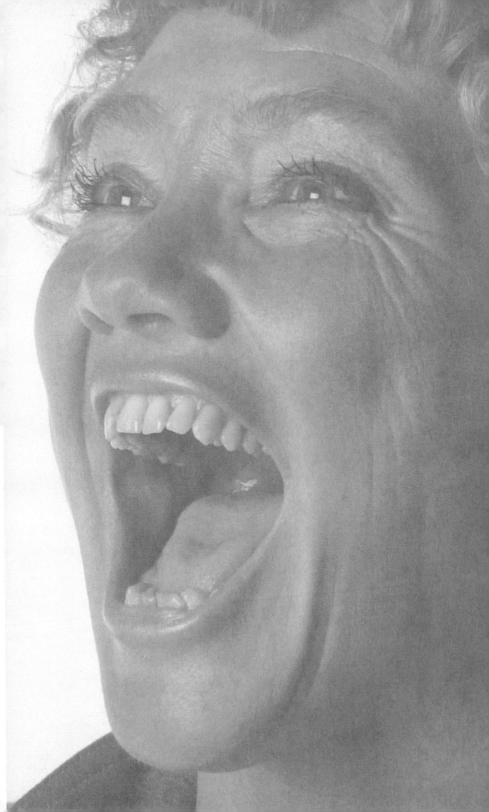

CHAPTER I

The Physiology of The Voice

Breath function

Every 4 or 5 seconds, we breathe. It is a vital and reflexive function, which operates whether we are aware of it or not, whether we are resting or sleeping, or performing a physical activity. Breathing is the body's most basic need. Without breathing, we would die.

We can only control our breathing to a certain extent. We can decide whether we will breathe quickly or slowly, lightly or deeply, or hold our breath—but only to a point. If we overdo it, our automatic control centre will take over.

The breathing organs include: the nose, mouth, larynx, trachea, bronchi and lungs.

When you breathe in, the breath passes first through the nose, where it is warmed, filtered, and moistened, so that the mucous membranes of the lungs receive it in the best way possible.

The path through the nose is significantly longer than that through the mouth. The nose is lined with tiny cilia, small hairs that remove dust, dirt and impurities from the air.

From the nose, the air passes through the trachea, which divides into two bronchi, each leading to one of the lungs. They divide further into a network of smaller tubes, called bronchioles, which terminate in small air sacs, called alveoli. The alveoli are surrounded by capillaries, which exchange oxygen and carbon dioxide in the blood.

The path of the breath

When you breathe in, the diaphragm—a large muscle located directly under the ribcage—contracts, causing the ribs to lift upward and outward. This increases the volume of the chest cavity. When you breathe out, the muscles relax again,

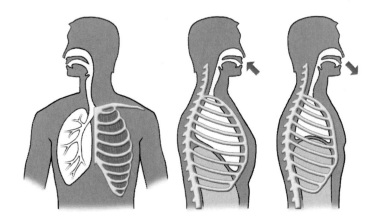

Fig. 1. The Lungs.   Fig. 2. Inhalation. Fig. 3. Exhalation

compressing the lungs.

The breathing muscles include the chest and shoulder muscles along with the diaphragm. As mentioned earlier, these muscles relax during exhalation. Imagine an inflated balloon leaking air. The exhalation during speaking and singing is based therefore on a muscular function in which the lungs' air capacity is decreasing.

The vocal cords sit inside the larynx and consist of mucous membrane-encased elastic bands. The glottis—the space between the vocal cords—can be opened and closed by contracting and relaxing the vocal cords. In a resting position—that is, when we are breathing and not speaking—the vocal cords are relaxed. The glottis is therefore open (Fig. 4). Here is missing a drawing of the open and closed glottis. When the glottis is closed, the vocal cords are contracted, as in speech or singing (Fig. 5).

When we speak or sing, the vocal cords are contracted, and air from the lungs passes through the narrow opening. The vocal cords vibrate, creating the sound.

The more forcefully the air is pushed through the opening, the louder the sound will be.

The opening between the vocal cords can be narrower or wider. This will cause the tone to be higher or lower.

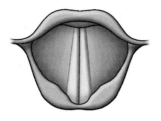 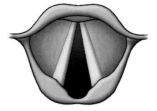

Fig. 4. Glottis closed.   **Fig. 5. Glottis open**

The individual's vocal range will depend largely on their physical characteristics, such as the shape of the mouth cavity, cheekbones, size of the tongue, and shape of the head.

The larynx

The larynx is a part of our speaking apparatus. It sits in front of the throat, and if you place your finger on it, you will feel it slide up and down as you swallow. If you hum with a closed mouth, you will also feel vibrations. The larynx should preferably be in a low, resting position when you sing or use your voice actively. You can train yourself to have this relaxed position in the larynx. During ordinary breathing, the larynx is open. In front is the trachea, and behind is the oesophagus. The epiglottis is a cartilage that closes over the trachea when you swallow, so that food doesn't go down the wrong way. The larynx is a vulnerable spot, especially because the trachea is so close to the skin.

It is interesting to see how animals in mortal danger expose the throat by throwing their head back in a sign of surrender, letting go of the last bit of control over their lives. There is an expression in Danish, *"med livet i halsen,"* or "with your life in your throat," which evokes the feeling of the larynx rising and blocking the flow of air when our life is threatened.

Resonance spaces

Everything vibrates to its own frequency. If we, for example, strike a wine glass, the tone we hear is its natural frequency,

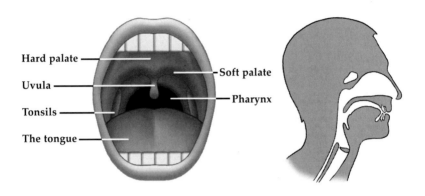

Fig. 6.   **Fig. 7. Resonance Cavities**

determined by the glass's size, shape and composition. If we can produce a tone with the same frequency, we can amplify the sound of the glass; if we make it louder and louder, the vibrations will be amplified so much that the glass will crack. We can therefore amplify and influence the glass's frequency from the outside.

If we enter a church, we will notice that the space amplifies certain sounds and tones. Some tones will be more apparent, and some will seem almost swallowed by the space. For example, there are some churches that seem to amplify speaking, and others that amplify singing. This is dependent on the size, shape and design of the church, as well as on what building materials were used. There is a huge difference between churches made of wood, and those made of stone or of glass. If we fill the room with furniture, carpets, or people, this will also influence the sounds we create in the room. By changing the space, we influence its ability to vibrate sympathetically with sounds. One might say that the way in which we change the space determines which kinds of tones will be amplified in it.

When we speak of resonance spaces in the body, we can understand them as our inner church space. We are born with a building we cannot change; with, for example, long legs, broad shoulders, short nose, small feet, etc. But when we speak of the voice, we actually have spaces we can change a great deal. The mouth cavity is the space we can change the most. With the help of tongue, lip, cheek and soft palate position, we can produce the sound we desire. The soft palate is like a sail between the hard palate and the uvula. Notice how the space in your mouth changes shape when you yawn, and the soft palate rises and sinks during inhalation and exhalation. Look in the mirror and open your mouth wide. You can clearly see the arch of the soft palate with the uvula hanging in the middle. Try to raise and lower the soft palate, as though you are yawning. You can also snort in and out and feel your soft palate tingle. This can be an effective way to relax a tense soft palate.

Among the most important spaces in which we can feel our voices resonate are the sinuses, not only those on either side of our nose, but also those above our eyebrows.

Voice and body type

As a rule, one would expect a direct relationship between body type and voice type—that is, a larger voice in a large body, and a smaller voice in a small body. When we see an elephant, we will automatically imagine a larger and rougher sound compared with a hummingbird. When we speak of the human voice, however, it is more complex. First and foremost, it is the size and thickness of the vocal cords that determine what kind of voice we have; but the shape of the head, the resonance spaces, and the way we use them also contribute to the voice's volume and unique qualities. Someone with a small body, strong vocal cords and excellent resonance spaces can have a voice that projects much farther than someone with a large body and weak vocal cords. We can train our voices and our vocal cords, and we can learn to exploit our resonance spaces, so that we can supplely change and adjust them according to our needs.

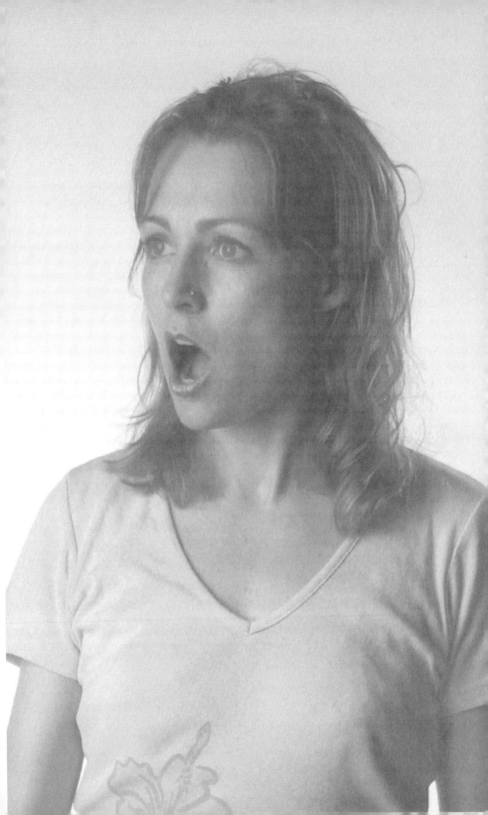

CHAPTER 2

Voice and personality

It's all hidden in the voice

"The telephone conversation left me completely confused. I could hear in his voice that something was terribly wrong. He sounded sad, not himself at all. At the same time he was telling me how good he felt, and how happy he was with his new job. I felt I could trust his voice more than what he was saying in words."

Your voice always paints a portrait of your immediate condition, here and now. It reflects your mood and your state of mind, how you react to internal and external influences. If you are depressed and unhappy, as in the above example, it is audible in your voice; likewise if you are angry and irritated. In other situations you may notice that your voice changes; it could for instance become smaller or disappear entirely, as in this example of a woman encountering a domineering colleague: "I could suddenly hear my own voice. Confronted by my colleague I nearly disappeared, and so did my voice. I became small and pleading, and had a hard time getting any words out." The situation reminds the woman of her relationship to her overbearing mother. The woman regresses, feeling small and oppressed, exactly as she felt early in her life.

Or, imagine that it was forbidden to express anger in your childhood home. In this case, since anger is a basic emotion, which must be given voice in order to be expressed fully, you cannot cope with anger in yourself or your surroundings—and it can be heard in your voice. Unexpressed anger is always audible. This is true of all the basic emotions. In order to feel we are whole and intact human beings, we must be able to express ourselves with sound. What is grief without weeping? Anger without shouting and screaming? Joy without cheers and

13

laughter?

When we begin to let our sound out—perhaps after years of disuse—we can be very surprised at the results.

One woman reports, "When I work with my voice, I can sometimes be astounded at how much sound and strength I have in me. I feel six feet tall and on top of the world."

Your voice can free you of so many obstacles that you actually get a physical boost, feeling taller and more expansive.

Even chronic conditions, mannerisms, habits and patterns in your voice acquired over time can be manifestations of unresolved episodes in your life; since you have not dealt with them or achieved some kind of closure, you carry them around with you—audibly. These may be expressed as tensions that can, for example, manifest as a chronic "cry" in the voice, or even a sensation of needing to clear your throat. What you really need to *clear* always has a story behind it, and pops up in situations that resemble what you once experienced.

You can work with the voice on many levels, depending on how deeply you would like to explore, and where you are in your life. The voice conceals its own "melodies," just as though it were an old-fashioned record player. Each record is engraved with a melody: an expression of some problem, theme or feeling in your life. The melodies on the records can be played one after the other, depending on where you are in your life and what you are ready to work with.

In this way, your voice is both a portrait of you here and now, playing the melody of the moment, and a sounding board, lending certain elements of your history, roots and background extra resonance.

More serious psychological or emotional traumas connected to crisis or shock can cause a temporary or chronic loss of voice, stammering, or vocal nodules and can lead to a loss of one's sense of identity.

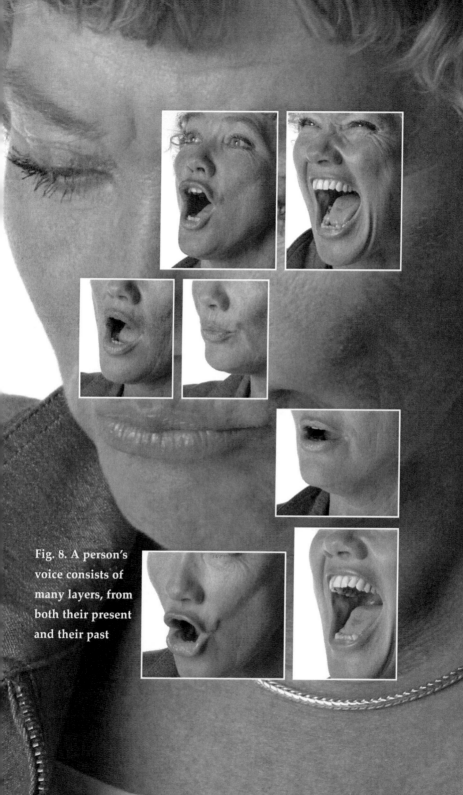

Fig. 8. A person's voice consists of many layers, from both their present and their past

Everything is made of sound

In the beginning, there was sound.

In the creation story in the first chapter of the gospel of John we hear, "In the beginning was the word. And the word was with God, and the word was God." Words and language are collections of sounds, to which we attribute particular meanings so that we can understand each other. The word "universe" (*uni versum*) means "one word." We might imagine that the entire universe consists of sound vibrations, pure and simple; said another way, everything is made of sound.

Non-Western cultures have known for millennia that sound can be used as a tool for healing or for altering consciousness. Sound—the voice—has been used as a means of achieving ecstasy along with ritual and religious purification, exemplified by Nada-yoga (the yoga of sound) in India. In this system, each sound frequency corresponds to one of the body's chakras.

Shamanistic ritual music, like the holy songs and dances of the Sufi and polyphonic songs from Tibet, also use sound and the power of the voice as a tool to achieve a higher state of consciousness.

Hans Jenny, a doctor and researcher from Switzerland, did ground-breaking work on the influence sound can have on material things. His experiments sent sound waves through media such as water, milk and sand. Different frequencies cause different shapes to manifest themselves as the media vibrate, and Jenny documented these forms with photographs. It turns out that the same shapes caused by the vibrations are also visible at a molecular level. Jenny believed that the key to understanding how we can heal the body with the help of sound lies in our understanding of how different sound frequencies can influence genes, cells and various structures in the body.

Sound can create harmony or chaos

Sound can create harmony or chaos. Sound can penetrate the

physical world. We are familiar with this from the Bible, in which Jericho's walls fell with the help of the trumpets' blast, and from the opera's prima donna, who shatters glass and mirrors with her high C.

These are two examples of how sound can influence material things if we can find the frequency that can crack walls or shatter mirrors. And if we can do that, it would certainly be thought-provoking if we could also repair walls or mirrors with the help of sound! In any case, we certainly experience both the positive and negative manipulation of sound in our daily lives.

It is possible to react so violently to loud or powerful sounds that you are physically affected, experiencing headache or other bodily discomfort. This could result from irritating mechanical sounds at your workplace, or a teenager's booming rock beats hour after hour.

We use the voice consciously or unconsciously in our daily lives, and we react to it as well. When a mother comforts her child after he falls and hurts himself, she uses her voice intuitively. She drops into a lower register, speaking more calmly and slowly, as if she is caressing the child with her voice. And the child calms down. The power of sound and voice can penetrate the filters of intellect and mind to reach deep reservoirs of emotion, provoking a physical reaction. For example, sound vibrations from a big city can directly cause pain, fatigue and nausea. But after coming home and listening to a CD with favourite songs, the physical discomfort can transform in just moments to bliss and well-being. The singing has restored harmony and balance.

Life begins and ends with sound

Just as it is said that the last thing to leave a dying person is their sense of hearing, it is the first breath, the first sound—the scream—that announces a human being's entry into this world. The breath is a sign of life. In the first months of life, a child is in constant contact with its sound, its voice. The voice is its most important tool for communicating the most basic needs: tenderness, love, contact and food. The voice is the child's fundamental means of communication, and more or less the only way it can as yet express pleasure or discomfort.

Later in its development, the child will embark on constant experimentation with its voice and its body in imitation of its surroundings, primarily its mother and father. In this phase, the child plays, explores, learns and experiments with its voice and body, and begins to self-identify. It seems that all movements have sound, and all sound is in motion. In this age, before language, it is unusual to see a child in motion without sound. Children can be heard, anything else is suspect; think of the mother who reacts immediately if she can no longer hear her child! Voice and body make up an elegant whole. The one cannot exist without the other.

The neglected voice

The child is a thing of perfection in sound and body, not yet burdened with a language.

It is when a child first acquires language that the division of head and body—that is, of intellect and emotion—begins. The child learns to communicate with words and no longer needs to express itself with body language and voice to the same degree. First the child learns to speak and walk—and then it learns to sit and be silent.

As the child grows, it is easier and easier to forget the body, the emotions, and the expression of the voice, especially if they are not constantly invoked. Parents, teachers and other authority figures teach the child to neglect the voice, also closing off inward perceptions and emotions in favour of more outwardly social behaviour. By saying this, I mean that the inner life is not taken as seriously as the outer. It is a much higher priority to teach the child to manage its daily tasks, that is, to conform itself to bound-

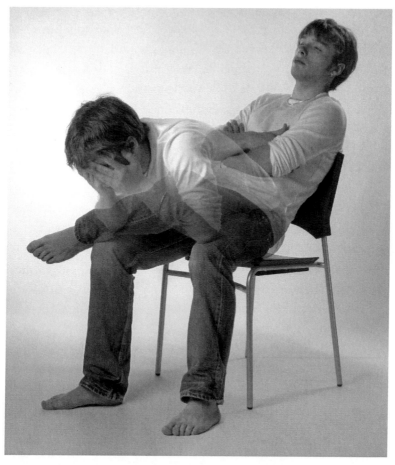

Fig. 9. What is on the inside is not always in harmony with what is on the outside.

aries and structure, obey collective instructions, cooperate with others, and to learn to read, spell, write and count. And even though these are important and useful, they unfortunately often come with a price: an amputated voice and amputated feelings, or a lack of contact with one's inner self. As an adult we may have to use time and energy trying to get in touch with this lost part. We say someone has "taken leave of their senses," to illustrate how lost we can become if we do not stay in touch with our inner and outer perceptions.

Many adults still discourage children's free expression with sound and have a relatively low threshold of tolerance. This may be connected to our difficulty tolerating others' (children's) sound, because it reminds us of all the sound we were obliged to silence in ourselves, and therefore cannot stand to confront. We set boundaries and rules for what the child may and may not do. For example, we teach them not to scream and shout "asshole" or "stupid idiot," when they need to blow off steam; but instead we teach them to control themselves and be rude in more hidden and indirect ways.

We have acquired language in order to better understand each other. But although we understand each other on one level, it is at the same time possible to misunderstand each other on other levels. We could say it another way: to have a language is also to be at its mercy. This means that we have acquired a tool to obscure and to distort reality. Through language, we are often deprived of our initial perceptions of the world and of our own reality.

A human being can communicate in more than one language and on more than one level, and is thereby able to send mixed messages.

We can therefore say one thing with words (verbally), and another, behind the words, with body language and intonation (nonverbally). It is important to be aware that children react spontaneously to what is being said with intonation and body language. They have a finely tuned perception, which is not yet spoiled by expectations, restrictions, or preconceived notions. For example, children will register a bad atmosphere between parents in an instant, even though it is not expressed in words, but only on non-linguistic levels. It is revealed in vocal range, intonation, and body language. Children are completely open to the present moment, and simply perceive the direct and obvious reality that we adults have forgotten or choose to deny because it does not suit us. An old saying goes, "children and fools speak the truth." The truth, then, is not limited by language, but is available to us if only we dare open ourselves and use our senses.

The essential stage in our development is to relearn how to sense with a child's clear attention, so we can achieve consistency between what we say and who we are. The goal must be to make our verbal and nonverbal expression not contradictory, but unified, so that our message as human beings can be heard as clearly and as authentically as possible.

Your voice is your calling card

No two voices are the same. The voice is like a fingerprint. It is your salient characteristic, your calling card. There are a multitude of different voice types, both speaking voices and singing voices. By your voice shall you be known. Let me hear your voice and I will tell you who you are. Your voice is both your singular feature and something that undergoes constant change. We use it differently depending on our mood and state of mind, and depending on whether we are speaking to our partner, our child, our boss, or our mother.

This is why an analysis of the voice and what it can tell us about a person can only ever be a snapshot and not a definitive judgement. We change all through our lives and have many different sides of ourselves that correspond to different periods in our lives. Still, there are consistent qualities or traits that characterise us more than others. These are perhaps clearest when those closest to us caricature us or otherwise make us aware of how we sound.

We can learn much when we listen to the voices in our day-to-day lives. The more we listen, the more we will come to know about the person in question and his or her way of living life. As we get better at listening to voices, we will note the different ways in which they are used, and how much they reveal. As mentioned before, there are no two voices that are alike, and no two voices that are used in the same way. The voice is a unique and precious instrument with which we share and express ourselves to the world around us. The voice reflects precisely where we are in the present moment. We can begin to take advantage of the possibility of listening to the voice behind the words, and above all trust the immediate experience of what we hear, applying our intuition. When we reveal our voices, we leave our calling card, as in the kind of situation where the sound of a voice still lingers in our awareness after the person has gone.

It is not really a question of using your voice correctly or incorrectly—that is, with respect to any rules. It is more a question of what we do and how we do it. Some people can talk for hours and leave their listeners breathless; others talk like a waterfall and bore their listeners to death. Some speak with an inner drive, and some with gentleness, while others speak in a monotone, or with melody in their voices. All of them affect us in different ways. Each person has his own, completely unique, ways of using his voice, and it is not a question of whether one is better than the other. We all have our reasons for using our voices as we do. If we become conscious of what we are doing and how we are doing it, we can choose to change our ways. When a voice is comfortable with itself and intriguing to hear, it is superfluous to judge it as right or wrong, good or bad.

We have a tendency in our society to judge and label each other. We judge each other by appearance; occupation; possessions such as house, car, boat and other status symbols; husband or wife, and his or her appearance; friends and acquaintances, and so on. With all these blanks to fill in, we often forget to live in the now. It is important to be able to face each other without prejudice and simply listen to voices. Then judgements become irrelevant, and the experience itself becomes important.

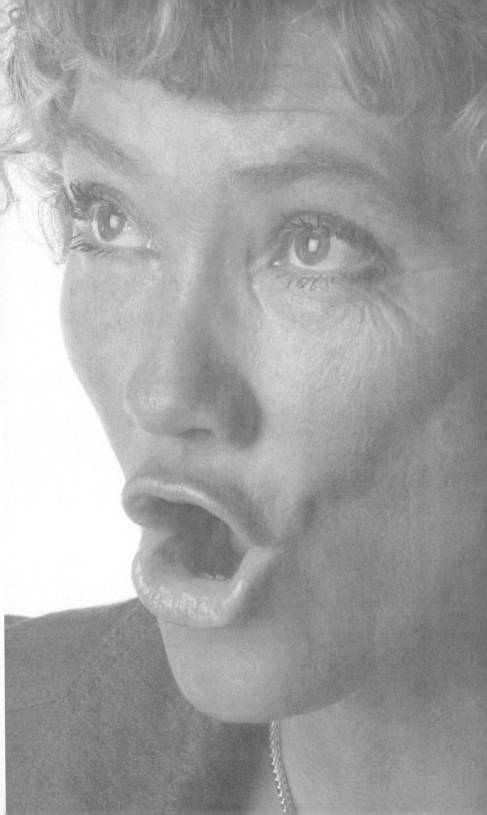

Chapter 3

The Raw Materials of the Voice

The chart below contains some of the most important components of the voice. I call them *the raw materials of the voice*. Each of these raw materials corresponds to a psychological characteristic. I hope above all else to demonstrate the connection that exists between the way we use our voice and the way we live our life. If, for example, we have a problem with the strength or volume of our voice, it could be that this is connected to our ability to make an impact generally. Have we lost strength in our voice because we are unable to exercise influence in our lives? Or the reverse? It's a chicken-or-egg question. It is therefore important to start seeing the voice as part of a larger whole, neither as something isolated, nor something we are born with and cannot change. When we are able to change our voice, a corresponding change will take place in our life.

The raw materials of the voice	What they reveal about our behaviour
Breath	Your ability to give and to receive
Sound	Your basic core, essence, identity
Strength	Your resources and ability to make an impact
Balance	The balance between your opposites (*high/low register, loud/soft*)
Comfort zone	The part of your range where you naturally speak or sing
Vocal line	Your direction and momentum, your *drive*

Breath

The breath is an essential and vital process, in which we give and take in a constant exchange between the external and the internal. This rhythm of breathing in and out is a fundamental pulsation, and reflects our patterns of rest and motion. A healthy and functional breath is a precondition of work with the voice. That said, we actually improve and regulate the breath when we work with the voice, as in singing. The natural breath is a breath that is balanced: the inhalation and the exhalation flow effortlessly and last the same amount of time. If we are under physical pressure, for example through exposure to a smoky room without enough oxygen, we react by becoming sluggish and sleepy, and we get out of balance. If we are under psychological pressure, for example because of stress, our breath will become choppy, shallow and irregular. If we are suddenly surprised, for example when we get a slight shock, we hold the breath for a moment, and the heart begins to pound. In other words, if our breath is disturbed, the whole human being gets out of balance. There are various techniques of breath therapy that can have supportive or healthful effects on the breath. For example, at times of intense emotional release, the breath can help the individual "come around" through deep and calm inhalation and exhalation.

The breath can be divided into four phases: an inhalation; a pause; an exhalation; a pause. The way you use these four phases in your breathing can reveal something about your life. The inhalation reveals something about your ability to receive. The exhalation reveals something about your ability to let go. In every single moment of our lives, we receive thoughts, feelings and actions from the outside world, while simultaneously we release thoughts, feelings and actions from our inner selves. The balance between the inhalation and the exhalation reveals something about the relationship between receiving and releasing in your life. For example, do you have difficulty receiving gifts, praise and recognition, and an easier time sacrificing yourself for others by providing and achieving for their sake? This will be familiar to many; we are raised in the mistaken belief that it is wicked to hoard too many good things for ourselves, but virtuous to be self-sacrificing. Your breath will reflect your relationship to these notions. The opposite is also possible, that your breath has too long an inhalation and too short an exhalation. This may mean that you take too much energy from other people. You may not be able to reject or filter the standards, demands or opinions of others. Said another way: you're not getting rid of what either isn't yours, or is of no use to you. Your breathing is a reflection of the eternal giving and receiving.

We must also pay attention to the two important pauses, since it is here we often prevent ourselves from letting our energy flow freely. That is, we either hold back the exhalation (so that we do not get rid of the air), or we hold back the inhalation (so that we do not take enough air in). In this way, many people develop a spastic tension that causes them to have difficulty releasing their exhalation. Also possible is the total absence of the two pauses, so that they rush along and do not get the full benefit from either inhalation or exhalation. There are countless variations to the way we breathe, and it is exciting when we begin to see the correlation between breath and lifestyle, and to make changes in both.

Example:

This example concerns a young woman. She uses a lot of energy in her exhalation, but does not get enough air when inhaling, leading to an imbalance in which she easily gets out of breath. Her way of breathing is just like that of an excited child telling a story: so excited, she forgets to breathe altogether.

She says that in her life, she has a tendency to give and give, and to push herself; but she has difficulty receiving, as well as difficulty listening and allowing herself the time and space to do what she really wants.

Sound

What is sound, exactly? We know the word from the world of music, when we say that music sounds good. Sound is a word with positive connotations, giving us a sensation of something grounded and strong. When we say that something is "sound," we are describing it as secure, healthy or well-built.

In music, we often describe sound as something that has a warm or cold "colour," or tone quality. We can talk about the voice in the same way. Ideally, a healthy sound is like a bell—brilliant and resonant. We can then go on to describe it based on its primary tone qualities. How we experience someone's tone quality is very personal, but there are general features that everyone agrees on. The tone quality of a voice is determined by, among other things, the shape of the mouth cavity, the size of the tongue, how we use our resonance spaces, and what inhibitions hold us back. All these factors contribute to why each person has her own unique tone quality, her own unique sound. The sound of the voice can reveal something about our innermost core, our essence. *Sound* in this respect has nothing to do with whether our voice is large or small, or whether we can use our vocal power or not; it has more to do with quality than quantity. For example, is the sound warm or cool, saturated or porous, sharp or soft, round or flat, open or closed? And yes, we quite simply have comparable traits in ourselves. For example, a woman whose voice has a warm sound is very often also a warm person. To achieve a healthy, authentic sound, we first have to work on ridding the voice of bad habits and inhibitions.

Sometimes we have to work to shed an excess of acquired technique. Those who have trained their voices for work within a particular musical genre often feel it is a huge job to unlearn these techniques.

They may have acquired a husky, airy tone appropriate to jazz style, or they may have sung with a compressed, pinched sound that would be ideal for certain kinds of rock music. This sound may even have become a kind of identity, but the authentic, pure and undisguised sound is often lost and must be found again by peeling multiple layers away. The original, authentic tone quality cannot be acquired by learning a particular technique, role or style; instead, we strengthen it by finding our way back to ourselves.

Example:

This example concerns a middle-aged man with a fairly closed and pinched sound. He has tensions in the root of his tongue, which cause him to sound like he has swallowed his tongue, or like his voice is wrapped in a blanket. In fact we cannot hear the sound of his voice properly, because there is something in the way. He will have to break through these barriers before his voice will resonate freely.

He explains that he has difficulty giving up control and expressing grief and sorrow in his life. Tensions in the root of the tongue are often expressions of control and can block a freely vibrating sound.

Strength

In some societies and families, there is such a taboo surrounding the use of the full volume of the voice that their members have gradually forgotten how to scream. Every healthy voice can scream—that is of course how all voices begin. Despite this, there are very few adults with an intact scream. It may be that most people associate a scream with fear rather than with joy. But screaming can just as easily be used to release our joy as to express our fear. It is a wonderful truth that the moment we choose to unleash our energy instead of holding it in, it automatically becomes something positive. Our strength is then accessible to us instead of opposed to us. Catastrophic thinking often prevents us from using the strength we have because we wrongly imagine it to be a kind of demon that possesses us.

There is a legend which says that evil is present only in that which is not revealed. It is inspiring to think that in the moment we unleash our energy, the darkness disappears. Most of us have much more strength than we think. We need only be willing to use it. We can use strength in two ways. In fact, all energy can go two ways, outward or inward. Either we use it outwardly, or it will turn inward against the self, where it can be destructive. Our strength, especially when manifested in anger, is an energy that can quite seriously take hold of us and cause illness if we constantly repress it. Instead, let it have free rein, so it can be transformed into the creative power it really is.

The strength in your voice is your volume. How much strength is there in your voice? How loudly can you shout or sing, when you use your full strength?

The power and strength of your voice always reside in your body. The better contact you have with your body, the more strength you will have.

Think of a situation in which you really must shout or scream—and you are leaning back comfortably in an easy chair. Presumably you would at the very least sit up and lean forward; and you would likely stand up completely in order to access your full strength.

It is mainly the diaphragm—your abdominal muscles—and your back muscles that you use when you turn up your volume.

When you have used your full strength, how do you sound afterwards? Are you hoarse because you have misused your power? This is just a sign that you don't use it enough; you have simply not learned—or you have forgotten—how to push that power button without abusing it. Imagine you are standing in a lecture hall, and that people all the way in the back row need to hear you. Breathe well and deeply and use your body; don't stand in one place. Allow yourself daily to exercise the strength in your voice. We have the strength, but it's no good to us unless we use it.

Example:

This woman feels powerless. She uses her power to deaden herself— that is, she turns her power against herself. This can be heard in the voice, which is squeaky, sobbing and pointed. She devalues her strength, dismantling it into melancholia. The "Poor Me" type is actually a tough cookie—a powerful person who has turned her strength upside down and in so doing manipulates her surroundings.

Balance

When we speak of balance, it almost always refers to the balance between two extremes, two opposites. When it concerns the voice, it can refer to the balance between high and low registers, or the balance between loud and soft notes. A voice in ideal balance can produce an even and free sound from one register to the other, easily shifting from high to low tones. Balance is also present when the voice can effortlessly shift from loud to soft. If any of these things is difficult, balance has not been achieved.

This is evidenced, for example, when there is no connection between two vocal registers. They function each in their own way and sound very different, as if the singer had two or more entirely different voices. Balance is also missing when a singer has no contact to his low register, for example, missing half of his voice. He may feel as if he has no depth at all.

Balance is about connecting these different voices, which correspond to different sides of our selves. They can be opposites: for example, masculinity and femininity.

First, contact must be re-established with the forgotten voices, and then they must be integrated in balance with each other. It is exciting and stimulating work.

Comfort zone

Your comfort zone is the pitch range in which you naturally speak or sing. It is where your voice functions best, sounds best, and has the most strength. It is where you belong, spontaneously and without special training.

The vocal range is divided into three registers: low (*chest voice*), middle (*middle voice*), and high (*head voice*). In addition to this there are the extra low (*vocal fry*) and the extra high (*whistle tones*) registers.

Example:

This woman has a good low register and correspondingly positive relationship to everything she associates with depth: "warmth, grounding, being direct, serious and authoritative." On the other hand, she has hardly any high register, and she has a negative relationship to what she associates with height: "shallow, hysterical, superficial and mock-feminine."

A challenge for her could be to transform her negative view of her high register to something more positive, for example, lightness, joy, spontaneity and femininity.

The world of music commonly divides the voices into soprano, alto, tenor and bass.

Soprano and alto are the high and low women's voices, respectively. Tenor and bass are the high and low men's voices.

Nature equips us with varying body types. Our vocal cords are also varied. The thickness and length of the vocal cords determine what kind of voice we have, or where our comfort zone lies.

With training we can extend our comfort zone far beyond

what nature has given us. You can also strengthen a particular register that otherwise is only weakly developed, or you can work to strengthen your entire vocal range.

Your vocal comfort zone corresponds to the sides of your self that you have the best contact with, and that are the most developed.

Example:

If you speak in too high a range, the voice will often sound shrill and give the impression of a lack of grounding and self-awareness. This could be a girl, who does not want to grow up—that is, an adult woman who is afraid to be who she is, and who plays at still being a girl. Or it could be a man who speaks in an unnaturally low range, thereby concealing or compensating for his hidden femininity.

Vocal line

Vocal line is the way you deploy your voice. You could also say it's the way you steer your ship, or navigate your life. How do you steer yourself? With what kind of motion do you go through life? The motion in your voice draws an arc in a landscape. Your vocal line can, for example, be stammering, freely flowing, or deadly monotone.

You can have rising or falling arcs, curls, sudden stops or accents. With your vocal line, you draw that landscape every time you open your mouth.

Is it full speed ahead, or a sudden slam on the brakes?

Is it a lively, curious, inquisitive stream that moves smoothly through the landscape, or is it a motion that lacks energy and struggles along?

The way your voice moves forward is aligned with the way you move through life: your direction in your life here and now.

It is your ability—or lack thereof—to tackle your life.

If you listen to this energy in voices, you will learn much about those around you.

Example:

This example is a man who speaks quickly with tremendous momentum. He stumbles over words and appears a bit hectic. In the course of only a few vocal exercises it becomes apparent that he has a tendency to stutter. He is, in fact, compensating for his stutter by trying to speak even faster. He shares that he feels as though he is constantly in a race with himself. He feels that everyone he meets makes demands on him, which he must meet. He basically needs to listen to what his stutter is telling him, and begin to take himself seriously.

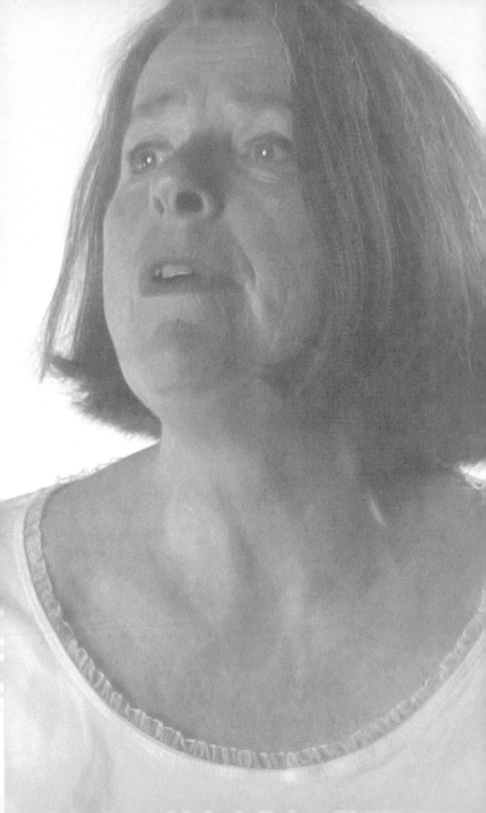

CHAPTER 4

Voice Types

What type am I?

All the voice types in the table on the following pages correspond to roles we play in our daily lives.

Behind these roles is the self, or the core. We could also call it the *real thing*. If we feel limited by the roles in our lives, and we don't achieve what we truly desire, we must take hold of these roles and work our way free of them. We need to discover and acknowledge which roles we take on, how and to what ends we use them, and when we set them aside. In this way we are able to make a conscious choice rather than being a slave to the role. We will also be able to achieve what we desire in a more honest way; this will afford us a more satisfying life, without the need to beg or otherwise manipulate others to get what we want.

When we are in dialogue with another person or persons, we react. The person we are facing affects us, and we may take on an amplified, extreme role. Depending on the situation we find ourselves in—a meeting with our boss, other authority figure, colleague, spouse, children, etc.—we will react in very different ways. We might be encouraged, angry, scheming, reserved, patronising, happy, emotional, witty, etc., in these encounters with others.

All these roles and expressions are also hidden in the voice. With the voice, we signal our state of mind and our reaction to what the other person is saying. A good listener can hear a lot in a voice, and is able to tell you who you are.

When we talk on the telephone, our hearing is sharpened, since our sense of sight is not in play. This means that the voice is in focus when we are on the phone. It is easy to pick up on what mood or condition those close to us are in, like our family or friends. Sometimes the words they say conflict with how they are saying them, and as a listener we can become confused by the mixed messages. Shall I listen for what you are saying with words, or what you are showing me with your voice? Which is truer, and how do I respond to what is being said?

Most of us have more than one role we play. That is, we have more than just our preferred voice, but rather a few that we can choose from in order to really get a result. Most of us are not only a "seducer" or a "little girl." In different situations, we use different masks, so most of us have a selection to choose from. We can develop many different roles and voices, and become good at them, just as an actor does. Which roles do you play? Which one is your favourite role, and what is that person like? We can become tired of our roles and masks, especially when we are trapped in them, and no longer feel we can freely choose when we use them and when we set them aside. To arrive at our true voice, we must first acknowledge our masks, and then choose to let them go.

How to identify your voice

How do I know if I sound like "The Wolf," "The Beggar," or "The Trombone"?

The first thing you can do is to become aware of your voice in all the situations you find yourself in from day to day. Ask those closest to you if they have noticed anything about how you sound. Spend time talking about the voice and how we usually use our voices, so you start to focus more on it. What others tell you about your voice can be a useful guide, but remember that only you can be your own judge; only you know what you are really feeling.

It is important to repeat that we do not have just one way of using our voices. We have many. The voice changes from situation to situation. Ideally, we should be able to freely switch between voices, fully aware of when we choose one or the other. But in order to do that, we need to know what our tendencies are.

We must become aware of which song we sing the most. How do we use our voice most often? Here are some key points you can try to be aware of in your communication with others, as you work towards finding out how you use your voice.

Energy

Notice if you have low energy or high energy. What is your first impression? Do you feel full of life and energetic, or sluggish and listless?

You might also feel ready on some days to take on the world and on others only fit to spend it on the couch. Evaluate yourself.

Types with high energy include The Wolf, The Starter, The Waterfall, The Seducer, The Beggar and The Trombone.

Types with average energy include The Echo, The Cocktail Party Voice, The Optimist and The Little Girl.

Types with low energy include The Pessimist, Hanging by a Thread, The Silent Voice, The Brake, The Control Freak, The Mumbler, The Hoarse Voice, Poor Me and The Killjoy.

Tempo

What are you most prone to: lots of speed, so that you almost trip over words? Or do you speak in a slow and relaxed tempo? Do you take pauses? Evaluate yourself.

Types with fast tempo include The Wolf, The Optimist, The Starter and The Waterfall.

Types with average tempo include The Echo, The Little Girl, The Trombone, The Mumbler, The Cocktail Party Voice, The Beggar and The Brake.

Types with slow tempo include The Pessimist, Hanging by a Thread, The Silent Voice, The Control Freak, The Hoarse Voice, Poor Me, The Killjoy and The Seducer.

Inflection

Notice your inflection. Does your voice have a tendency to go up or down in the course of a sentence? Or do you tend to stay in the middle? This is often revealed by the very last word or syllable in a sentence. Evaluate yourself.

Types with rising inflection include The Optimist, Hanging by a Thread, The Little Girl, The Cocktail Party Voice, The Beggar and The Seducer.

Types with a moderated inflection include The Echo, The Waterfall, The Mumbler and The Silent Voice.

Types with a falling inflection include The Wolf, The Pessimist, The Starter, The Brake, The Control Freak, The Trombone, The Hoarse Voice, Poor Me and The Killjoy.

Familiarity or distance

You can easily tell when you have really good contact with another person and feel secure with them. Your voice can reflect that trust and intimacy, for example, when you are with a good friend or your partner. When you have greater distance in your voice, you may speak like a narrator, lecturer, receptionist or sales clerk. The voice in this case sounds farther away and less personal. Evaluate yourself.

Types with familiarity in the voice include The Wolf, The Optimist, The Starter, Hanging by a Thread, The Echo, The Little Girl, The Trombone, Poor Me, The Beggar, The Seducer and The Hoarse Voice.

Types with distance in the voice include The Pessimist, The Starter, Hanging by a Thread, The Waterfall, The Silent Voice, The Brake, The Control Freak, The Mumbler, The Cocktail Party Voice and The Killjoy.

When you have identified which sides of your voice you know and use the most, you will quickly be able to move on to the table and start to recognise the different voice types. It is important at this stage that you do not judge yourself too harshly. Everyone has some of these qualities in them. Look upon yourself with a loving eye.

Important! This table is not a classification of people or an attempt to brand them. It should be understood and used as a stimulus to reveal certain patterns in voice and behaviour.

We have many different facets and use several of these voice patterns every day, so you can easily be several types at once. There is nothing wrong with that. It is only when you use one pattern exclusively—hardening into one voice type or behaviour—that there are grounds for concern. Variety is the spice of life.

Name	Voice Type	Behaviour	Question	Exercises
The Wolf	Attack in the voice	Attacks the whole world	Who or what are you defending yourself against?	Defence exercise
The Optimist	Rising inflection	Lets too much of the outside world in	Who or what do you resist saying no to?	Boundary exercise
The Pessimist	Falling inflection	Lets too little of the outside world in	Who or what do you resist saying yes to?	Release-the-energy exercise
The Starter	Energy at beginning of sentences	Open and present at first, but later withdraws	What happens if you hold yourself back?	Steady Energy exercise, grounding
Hanging by a Thread	Energy at ends of sentences	Not attentive and present until the end	What happens if you go first?	Charge exercise
The Echo	Variable voice	Echoes others, adapts, goes along	What are you avoiding?	Say-no exercise
The Waterfall	No pauses, lack of exhalation	Nervous and insecure, drowns out others and self	Who doesn't want to hear you?	Stop, Look and Listen exercise

Name	Voice Type	Behaviour	Question	Exercises
The Silent Voice	Quiet or no sound at all	Holds back much. The silent treatment, perhaps?	What is in an empty space?	Fill-the-space exercise
The Brake	Interrupted, stuttering	Tense and frustrated-sounding inflection	Who or what do you resist spitting out?	Take-what's-yours exercise
The Control Freak	Tension in root of the tongue	Lack of affection	Who or what is controlling you?	Surrender exercise
The Little Girl	High-pitched speaking voice	Lack of grounding	What do big girls do?	Sensation exercise
The Mumbler	Swallows words, speaks with unclear and tiny voice	Lack of self-worth and confidence	What do you accept without questioning?	Spit-it-out exercise
The Trombone	Speaks with exaggerated voice, continuously and without listening	Feels small and overlooked	Whom or what are you trying to drown out?	Make-space exercise
The Cocktail Party Voice	Sounds peripheral, as though not in contact with the body	Not in contact with feelings	Whom are you trying to satisfy?	Predator exercise
The Hoarse Voice	Vocal cords do not fully close	Seeks attention	Whom do you wish would hear you?	Singing exercises
Poor Me	Whimpering, sighing and whining in the voice	Asking for help from the world around	Whom do you need to help?	Bragging exercise
The Killjoy	Flat, pressed and withheld voice	Uses energy to hold self and others back	Who is squeezing the life out of you?	Champagne exercise
The Beggar	Flattering voice	You can't resist me	What do you want?	Dictator exercise

Name	Voice Type	Behaviour	Question	Exercises
The Seducer	Intimate, sensual and seductive voice	Seduces and manipulates others	How do others seduce you?	Cool-off exercise
The Throat-Clearer	Clears throat and coughs. Seems uncertain, arrogant and scolding	Has a chronic frog in the throat	What is it you're not able to say?	Sing-your-throat-clear exercise

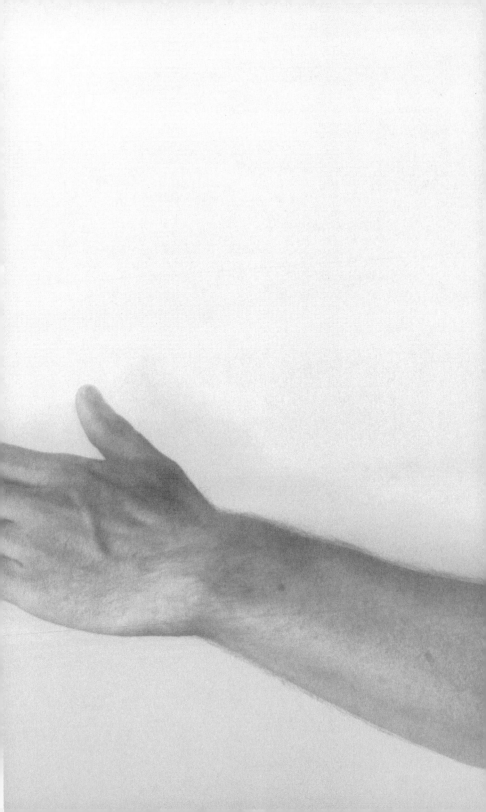

CHAPTER 5

Basic Exercises

Train your voice daily by listening to it and being aware of it. Record yourself, preferably while talking with other people, so you can get used to hearing what you sound like.

Read aloud from books you enjoy, and practise various kinds of expression with your voice.

Stand in front of a mirror and watch yourself as you speak and sing.

You will frequently be surprised by these encounters with yourself. Do I really sound like that? Is that what I do?

Ask a few good friends to describe your voice for you in a loving way. Each piece of feedback will be helpful as you gain greater insight into both how you use your voice and how you understand yourself.

Introduction to the basic exercises

It is a good idea to begin each day with basic exercises. Take just one each day to start with, until you feel entirely comfortable with it. If you are able to dedicate more time, you can of course try them all; but in my experience you will get more out of learning one in depth than trying several more superficially.

Vocal shake

This exercise is a good one for warming up and for releasing excess control. You can also clearly hear and feel where along the scale you are comfortable and where you have problems.

Stand with your feet well apart but parallel to one another.

Notice the balance in your body by shifting your weight from your left foot to your right. Keep the ball of your foot in contact with the floor while you alternately lift your left and right heels.

Imagine your inhalation all the way down in your feet.

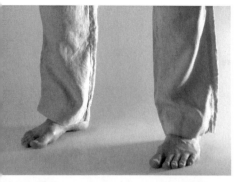

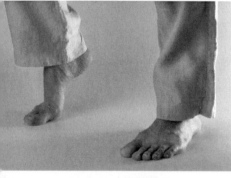

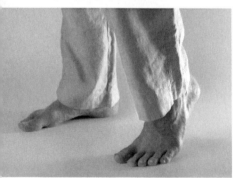

It is important to focus on the weight of your body, and feel that all your joints are soft and mobile; that is, the joints are neither tense nor overextended.

Begin slowly by bringing your breathing and your voice into the rhythm of your feet, like a train getting started. Gradually increase the tempo until your whole body is shaking.

Always envision the sound coming from below: up and out.

The Elevator

This exercise is good for checking your various registers: your low, middle and high voices. There ought not to be gaps in the voice; in other words, it should not crack or break at any point. This is a sign of a lack of connection to or contact with the body.

Stand well with an open posture.

Imagine that your body takes up a great deal of space, and there is plenty of room both inside and outside of your body.

Begin a tone as low as possible on an [ah] or [oh] vowel.

Now glide slowly up, and allow yourself time to breathe along the way.

At the same time, move your body in your own rhythm, as though you are painting or sculpting the sound.

As you come up into your higher register, change the vowel to

[oh] and then [oo].

Make space for the high notes, releasing rather than pushing them.

Vary the tempo as you please.

You can also try this exercise using a lip flutter or tongue trills, in order to relax these muscles.

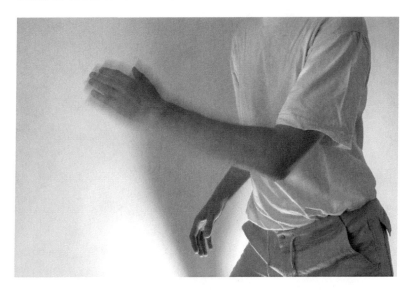

The Samurai

Many people have power and strength, but are either afraid to use it, or tend to abuse it by, for example, turning it against themselves. This exercise will help you turn your strength outward and can give you better alertness, energy, centring and joy.

Begin with your feet. Stomp on the floor for a while.

Use your entire body, so that you are really standing on your feet, and ground yourself.

Begin making any sound you like, and using your body.

Use your arms and hands to create boundaries around yourself, as if you held two swords slashing through the air.

"Chop" with your right arm at the same time as you stamp

with your left foot, and vice versa.

Move around the room like an angry samurai.

Use your voice in different ways, emphasising consonants.

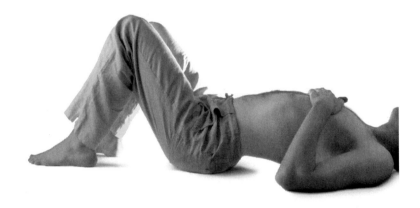

The Deep Breath

This exercise is fundamental and should probably be the first thing you do when you decide to work with your voice. It will help you to achieve a low inhalation, and can liberate a lot of life energy in your pelvic area. It is especially good if, for reasons of stress, nervousness or fear, your breath is too short or too high.

Lie on your back with your knees bent and the soles of your feet on the floor.

Breathe in as deeply as you can, and arch the small of your back enough so that you can fit your hand between your lower back and the floor. Breathe out slowly and calmly, as you press your back towards the floor and lift your buttocks upwards, free of the floor.

On the exhalation you may add a variety of sounds:

1. Voiced consonant like [z].
2. A low humming sound with closed mouth like [mm].
3. A low note on a vowel like [ah].

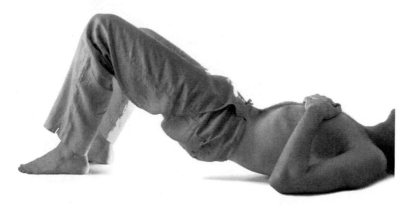

By adding sound to your exhalation you can more easily observe it and be aware of it.

Try taking time with your exhalation. How many seconds does it last?

Design your own programme

Generally these basic exercises are useful as a warm-up and can be combined with exercises for your particular voice type. You can also organise the exercises entirely according to your own needs and how much time you have. Here is an example of a daily programme:

Morning	Afternoon	Evening
Basic exercises:		Basic exercises:
Vocal shake, Elevator	Exercises for your voice type	The Deep Breath
	(*for example, The Beggar*):	
	Dictator exercise, Protest songs	

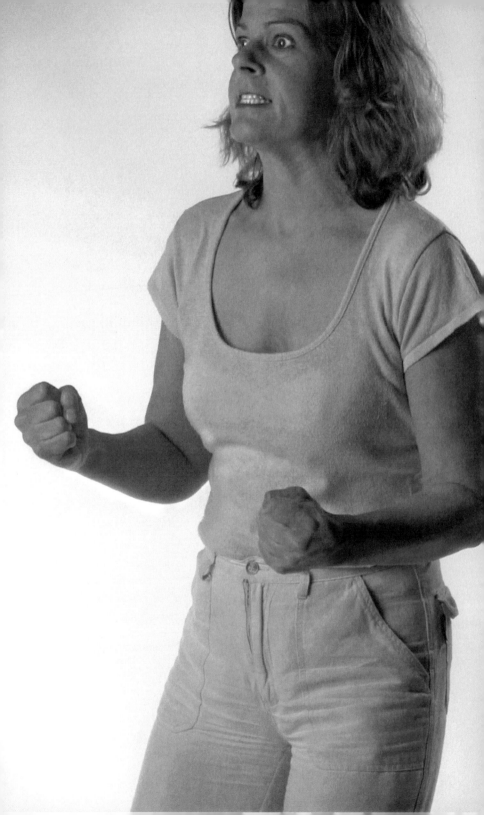

CHAPTER 6

Exercises for Your Voice Type

In these simple exercises you will have to take yourself seriously and not worry about decorum. Some of the exercises here might require you to step outside your boundaries, but they should at the same time cause you to smile; there is joy and vitality in them if you dare to invest yourself fully in them. You will have to silence your inner judge, who will tell you that you look completely foolish, or that there is something seriously wrong with you. To make it easier, try to have a childlike, playful spirit; the exercises will have a contagious, gripping, and redemptive effect on your surroundings. Just try! Even though they are intended for different voice types, you can get something out of each and every one, and they will lay a good foundation for your vocal training. You can also use them with a partner or with your family.

How often?

As a rule it is the case that you should practise as often as possible in order for the exercises to have the desired effect. The best outcomes result from doing them for a short period of time, several times a day, for example for 3-5 minutes, 3-4 times daily.

When?

Immediately before an important conversation, meeting or lecture, in which you predict you may have problems with your voice; beyond that, as often as you have the inclination and the opportunity to practise.

Important note

In each description of the different voice types, you will read the pronoun "he" or "she." This is only for ease of reading; every voice type is present in both men and women.

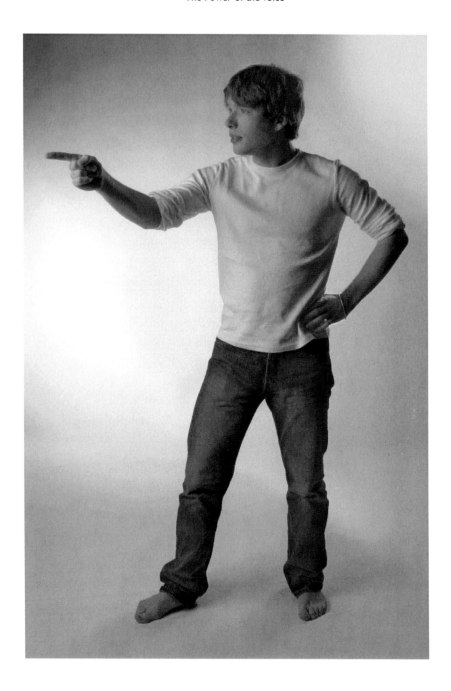

The Wolf

Description

The Wolf attacks with an aggressive glottal quality in the voice, and often speaks quite quickly. We all have a bit of The Wolf in us when we are angry. When you hear a Wolf voice, you might feel put down or even assaulted. Often The Wolf will paralyse his victim; that is to say, he or she is silenced in one way or another. For example, I once heard a Wolf give a lecture; it was remarkable that no one asked any questions afterwards.

Explanation

In reality, the impassioned attack of The Wolf is really a defence mechanism. Often, The Wolf is actually extremely vulnerable and insecure, and may himself have been the victim of attack. He is in that sense a hunted animal—a hunted person—who in turn hunts everything around him. Many politicians are Wolf types.

Solution: Defence exercise

Move slowly around the room, almost in slow motion. Breathe deeply and slowly. Be ready, on your guard. Imagine you are Peter Sellars in *The Pink Panther*, constantly defending yourself from the surprise attacks of your faithful servant Cato. Stop suddenly and deflect a blow, as though you were being attacked. Use your arms to defend yourself from the invisible enemy as you shout Ha! or Hoo!

Songs for your type

Religious songs, children's songs

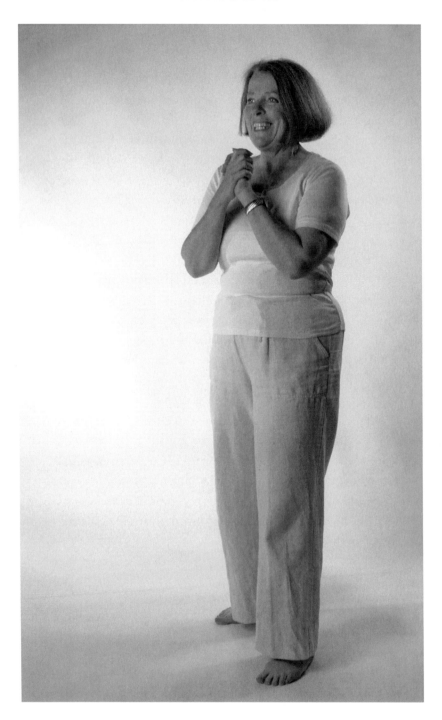

The Optimist

Description

The Optimist has a rising melody in her intonation and often speaks in a high register. Sometimes there is almost laughter in the voice. This is a person who can spread happiness and energy wherever she goes. There can be a tendency, though, to exaggerate the optimism so that it becomes a cliché: "Aren't we having fun?"

Explanation

The Optimist is clearly afraid of her less-acknowledged feelings like anger, grief and sexuality, and protects herself with an exaggerated happiness. There is also a tendency to blend into the background, and therefore a need for clear boundaries between self and surroundings.

Solution: Boundary exercise

Stand in a spot with plenty of room around you. Imagine now that you need to build a house around you. A boundary house, or your own personal and private space. What will it look like, and what materials is it made of? Give yourself plenty of time, and build it with sound, as if you were drawing or painting with sound.

Songs for your type

Protest songs, working songs

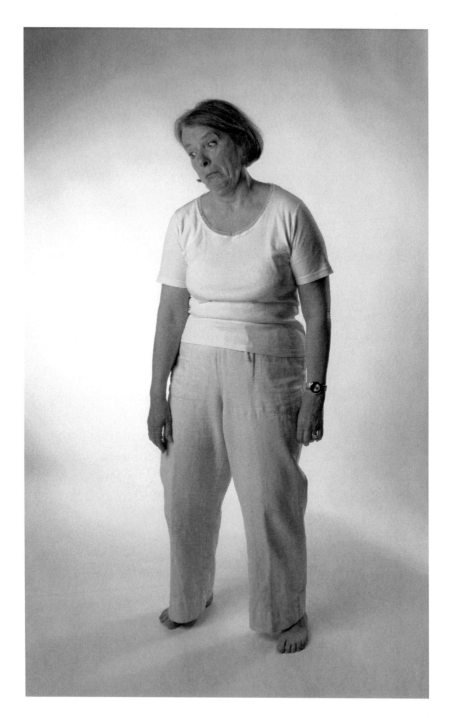

The Pessimist

Description

The Pessimist speaks with a quiet voice and falling intonation, at times in a slow tempo, at times "swallowing" the last word in a sentence. As the name suggests, this is a person who has a tendency to focus on the negative, worrying and complaining. She lacks confidence in herself and her surroundings and dwells on her own misery.

Explanation

The Pessimist is a person who probably has unresolved grief or pain in her. In the attempt to survive, she has turned that energy on herself, blaming and tormenting herself with reproaches and destructive self-criticism.

Solution: Energy-release exercise

Imagine that you are holding a ball that you want to slam into a net. Run around a little with the ball. Do it with sound, and use your whole body. Take a running start. Say [ah-ee] or [ah-oo]. On the [ee] and [oo] take your shot, allowing your voice to glide up. Make sure you release your voice in the high register, so the shot is really delivered.

Songs for your type

Hymns of thanksgiving and joy, ballads, heroic songs

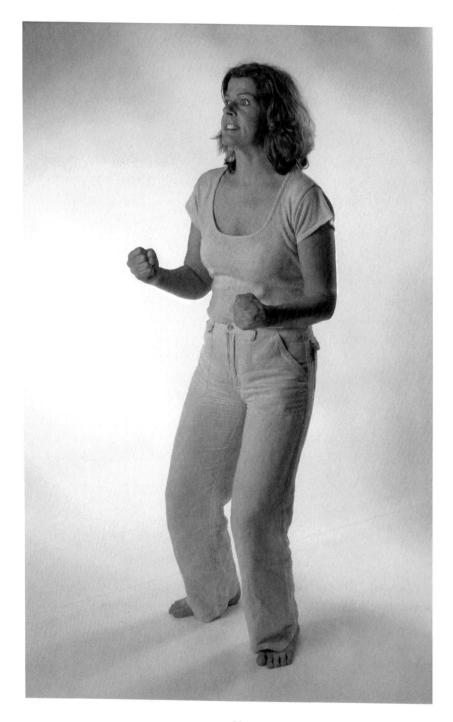

The Starter

Description

The Starter is a person who burns off all his energy before he even gets in the door. This type speaks quickly, loudly and clearly, and there is a strong presence and engagement in the voice from the first second.

The energy dissipates quickly, however—the air goes out of the balloon, as it were—and after a while the tempo becomes quieter, and the intonation more muted.

Explanation

This is a type that feels pressured to accomplish a great deal and to live up to high expectations. So much energy is invested in the beginning of a meeting with others that there is a tendency to become completely exhausted and borderline discouraged. Therefore it also becomes difficult to deliver on what he has promised. This is a person who may not yet have freed himself from others' expectations; in any case, there is a need to economise on energy or hold some back.

Solution: Steady Energy Exercise

Take any book at random, and stand with feet parallel and lightly bent knees. Begin your reading softly and calmly with a quiet voice. Read aloud in an evenly flowing tempo. Be sure to use your air until you have no more air remaining. Hold on and follow through completely in your sentence. You may also choose to speak a stream of nonsense words, but that may demand a little more courage.

Songs for your type

Hymns, love songs, funeral songs

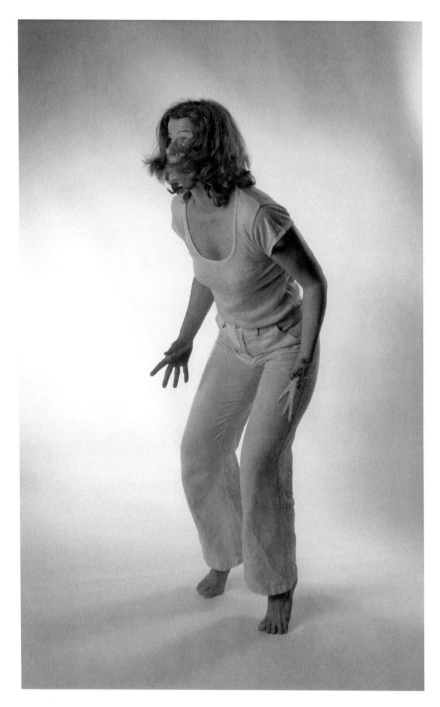

Hanging by a Thread

Description

If you wait long enough, you will eventually meet this type of person. The energy of the voice doesn't arrive until the end of a sentence or a conversation. It is quiet and withheld, often pitched low, and then suddenly clear and powerful. This is often a person who observes situations and people before throwing herself into a new enterprise, like a cat who waits a long time before pouncing. On the other hand, once she has taken on a project, she is very stable.

Explanation

"Once bitten, twice shy." This type has probably experienced hard knocks, involving pain and disappointment, which get in the way of more spontaneous behaviour. Perhaps she is even tormented by catastrophic thinking or danger fantasies about what can happen when she is spontaneous, which unconsciously make her afraid of trying new things.

Solution: Charge! exercise

Stand a little away from the centre of the room. Use the Samurai exercise (see description in Chapter 5). Imagine that your opponent is in the middle of the room, so your attacks always move you to the centre. Focus directly on your opponent and practise charging him again and again.

Also, practise getting straight to the point when you are with other people. Prepare your message (which can be super-short), and practise being direct.

Songs for your type

Drinking songs, sea chanteys, wedding songs, songs of rejoicing

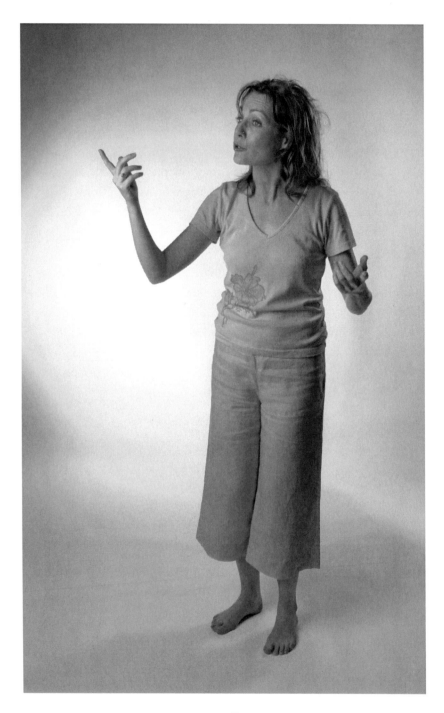

The Echo

Description

The Echo changes register, tempo and volume according to his surroundings, and is a master of adaptation in every situation. The Echo imitates and mimics his surroundings just like a small child copying mummy and daddy. It is therefore common to feel immediately at home with and understood by an Echo-type. This is a person that can change his voice as quickly as the mood strikes him. The typical Echo is a kind of yes-man, who lacks independent opinions.

Explanation

The Echo does not dare to come in real contact with himself for fear of being rejected. He avoids confrontation and achieves false contact with others by adapting himself to the situation. The Echo probably learned to adapt early on in life in order to avoid conflict and to obtain acceptance and love from his parents.

Solution: Say-no exercise

Stand up, breathe deeply and feel your feet in contact with the floor. Now exercise your power by saying "No!" while simultaneously stamping on the floor and striking out with your arms. It is important that you can feel your whole body working. Also use nonverbal sounds like [mah], [nah], [kah], [sah], using an open [ah] vowel as in *father*. You can also explore in order to find your own sounds, your own power.

Songs for your type

Protest songs, working songs, football songs

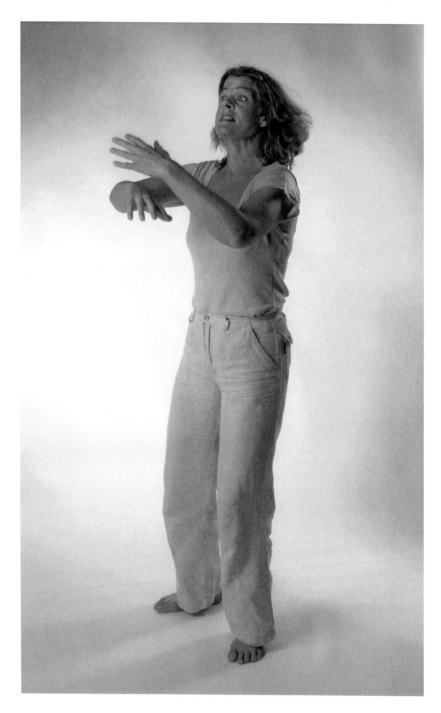

The Waterfall

Description

The Waterfall talks constantly and without pause, most often in a high register. She talks her way out of the heart of the matter, away from confronting her own feelings. This type is also prone to talking to herself, as if to avoid silence. We all know this type, able to speak for hours, even though she has long ago lost her listeners. As a listener, you get the feeling that your presence or absence is immaterial.

Explanation

The Waterfall uses her talking to avoid something else. She simply does not listen to others. When you speak so excessively, you keep yourself and others busy and avoid real contact; it is, then, a method of holding others at a distance. The Waterfall is in reality nervous and uncertain, afraid of her feelings and of the reactions of others. Perhaps this is a person who was herself held at a distance by one of her parents. Behind The Waterfall's uncertainty there can be strong, hidden feelings of grief and anger.

Solution: Stop, Look and Listen exercise

Stand with parallel feet and bent knees. Give yourself time to be aware of your body. Now read from any text in a very calm tempo. Take a pause after each sentence. Breathe and feel what happens to you and your body. When you have done this for a while, begin taking a pause after each word. Let the word resound fully, and notice again what happens. What are you using your pauses for? When you talk to other people, practise taking pauses. Use your breathing when taking a pause, and give yourself time to breathe in and out.

Songs for your type

Intimate songs, love songs, lullabies

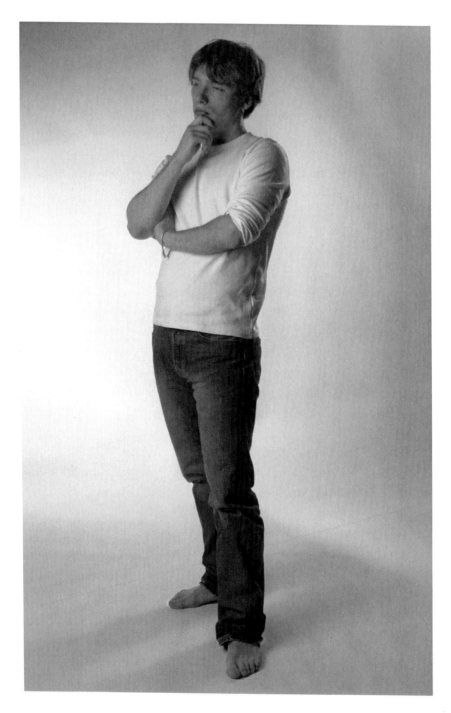

The Silent Voice

Description

It is obviously difficult to get an impression of The Silent Voice type, since there is so rarely any sound. Still, silence can be among the most eloquent types of expression. Silence can be an expression of something being held back; it can express both agreement (what we call *tacit consent*) and disagreement.

Explanation

When you use silence to hold something back, you are able to control and manipulate more than even you may be aware of. By not communicating where you stand and what you think, you can indirectly obtain quite a lot of power. So, silence can be a way of holding back in order to not lose that control, or it can also be used to punish—what we call giving someone the silent treatment. At bottom, The Silent Voice is perhaps a person who has become very disappointed and disillusioned in his life, and who hides hurt feelings.

Solution: Fill-the-space exercise

Imagine yourself in a huge empty space. What would you like to fill it with? Use your imagination. Now imagine that you will fill the space with sound. Fill that space with all the sounds you can think of: baby sounds, four-letter words, beautiful songs, terrifying shrieks, etc. You choose.

When you are silent when in contact with other people, what happens to you then? Try to be aware of your feelings.

Songs for your type

All kinds of songs

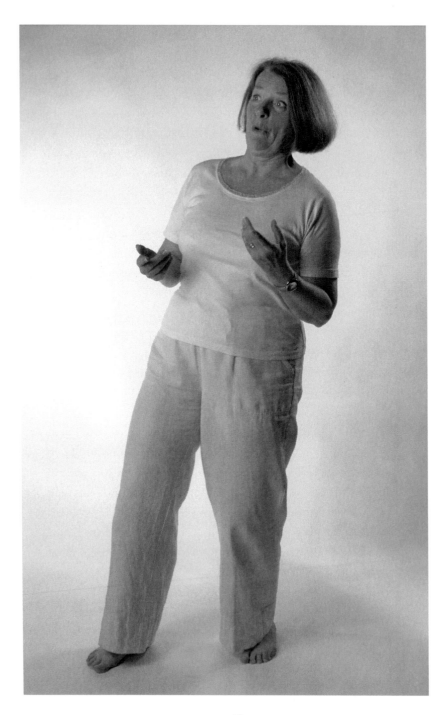

The Brake

Description

The Brake is known for an interrupted and stuttering intonation, as though there is some kind of inner brake being applied all the time. Some of this type stop in the middle of a sentence and do not complete it. Others stop, and then complete the sentence, but with stammers and breaks that make it hard for a listener to stay focused for very long. The voice is in an average register, but it is troubled by inhibited breathing, causing it to sound tense or frustrated; hoarseness, tension, and frequent throat-clearing can result. The Brake is exhausting to listeners.

Explanation

The Brake may have been stopped earlier in his life in a situation where he wanted to express himself. That is, he was prevented from fulfilling a need, and the situation has stuck to his voice on a psychic level. He then continues to stop himself from getting his needs met (for example, the need to express himself freely).

Solution: Take-what's-yours exercise

Imagine you are a very greedy person. Move around the room while you demand and greedily reach out for different objects. Take them by the armful. Use your imagination, thinking, "I want it all." Do not take any pause, but rather continue to free-associate.

Also try to be aware of what causes you to stop in the middle of a sentence when you are with others. What thoughts or feelings do you have?

Songs for your type

Civil rights songs, drinking songs, sea chanteys

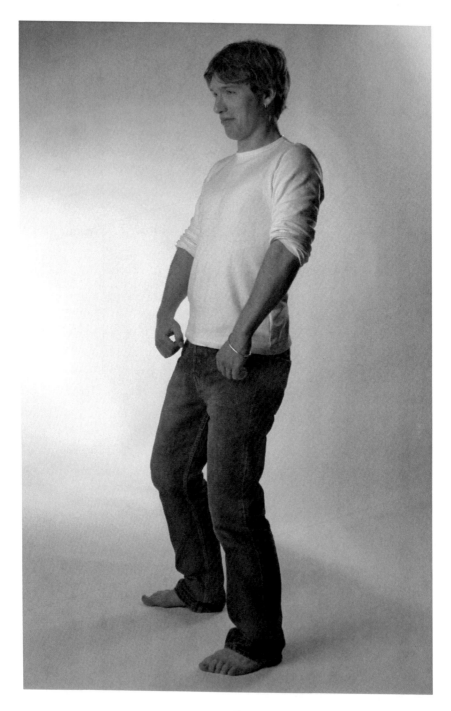

The Control Freak

Description

The Control Freak speaks with tension in the root of the tongue: that is, the tongue slides back in the mouth, where it blocks the free motion of air, and the voice sounds squeezed, as though she had a potato in her mouth. The tongue is known to have a relationship to control. The Control Freak's vocal comfort zone is probably slightly or very low. She desperately needs to control herself and the world around her. This is accomplished by holding back energy, and not stepping forward; we control by holding back. In a group setting, The Control Freak might work against suggestions either by passively dodging or actively opposing them. She controls by sabotage, and can poison any good atmosphere.

Explanation

The Control Freak has difficulty giving herself over to life, and uses control to get the attention she longs for, even if it is negative attention. This type exerts special control over her anger and grief, thereby punishing those around her and herself instead of showing her feelings directly.

Solution: Surrender exercise

Allow yourself to be completely foolish. Speak like a drunk. Let the words glide up and down, loud and soft, completely uncontrolled. Exaggerate this. Act really crazy. You can also choose a song and sing it as terribly as possible; this will really give you energy.

Songs for your type

Erotic songs, drinking songs, sea chanteys

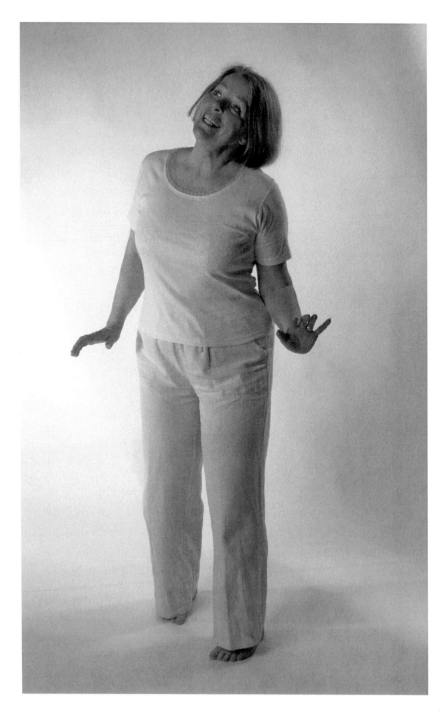

The Little Girl

Description

The Little Girl speaks, as the name implies, with the voice of a young girl. The register is high, and the voice is thin, weak or shrill. Sometimes The Little Girl can sound innocent or meek as a lamb. She hands over responsibility to others.

Explanation

The Little Girl certainly achieves a great deal by speaking as she does, but when women of a certain age persist in speaking like a little girl, something is wrong. This is a sign that she is afraid of growing up and taking responsibility. As a rule she insists on remaining in an old role, and she may have many reasons for this. The essential point is that she either does not dare feel and take seriously signals from her own body, or perhaps does not dare to acknowledge her body at all.

Solution: Sensation exercise

Begin by being aware of your feet and legs. Stand and kick a bit and shake them loose. Then begin rocking your hips in a smooth motion, like a belly dancer. Now use your low voice on a vowel like [ah] or [oh], and sing a song you know well. Make it into a charming and seductive song.

Songs for your type

Protest songs, erotic songs, football songs

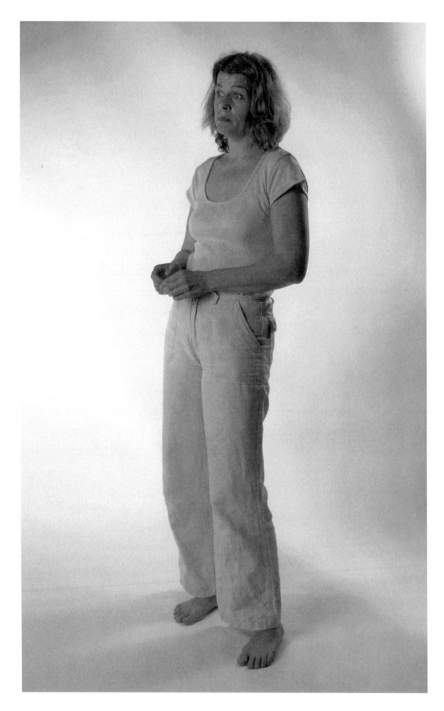

The Mumbler

Description

The Mumbler speaks unclearly and imprecisely, with a weak voice, in a medium or low register. Most often the listener must struggle to hear and understand what is said, and can easily become irritated. The Mumbler therefore typically gets a negative reaction to his speech.

Explanation

The Mumbler is often insecure and shy. This is a type who seems to apologise for taking up space, and lacks self-confidence. The Mumbler makes himself smaller than he is, and is constantly reinforcing his negative pattern: if he continues to get negative responses from others, then he must be worthless. This is definitely a person who has met rejection or anger from his parents, and continues in his mumbling voice to apologise for his existence.

Solution: Spit-it-out exercise

Begin by stretching, and take a few deep breaths; focus on exhaling the breath completely. Take any book and begin reading aloud. Articulate each and every sound extremely clearly, and do this with increasing volume. Next, make a list of swear words, including the worst words you know. When you have written them all down, stand up and begin spitting them out. Use the power of your voice and shout them with clear articulation.

Songs for your type

Recitatives, heroic odes, hymns, ballads, military songs

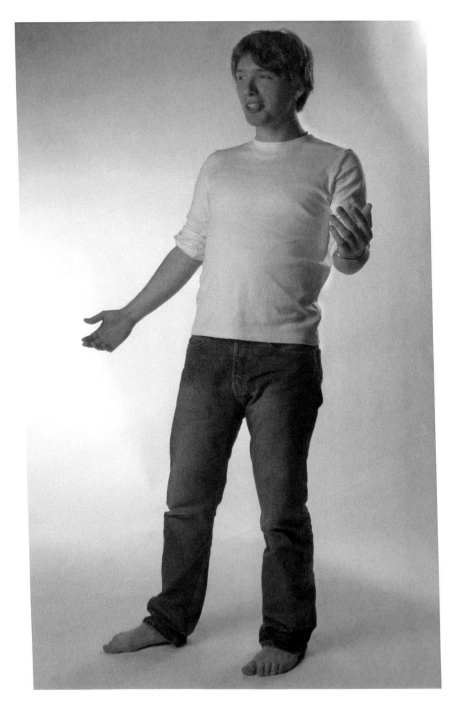

The Trombone

Description

The Trombone speaks forcefully in an average or high register. This type is easily picked out of a group, since he is often the only one who can be heard. The Trombone has a tendency to exaggerate just about everything, and if someone tries to interrupt, he just speaks louder. His weak spot is that he is not in contact—that is, in reality, there is no dialogue happening. The Trombone is alone on the stage and speaks too loudly and too long, without ever listening.

Explanation

The Trombone is similar to The Waterfall. In truth, he feels small and overlooked. But The Trombone is angrier and more stubborn, whereas The Waterfall is a more nervous type. The Trombone has himself been drowned out, and is now taking revenge in his own aggressive way. He gets rid of much of his angry energy by steamrolling everyone in his way, but rarely achieves a fruitful and sharing contact. The Trombone drowns out others, but also himself and his deeper feelings.

Solution: Make Room exercise

Make your voice childlike. Try copying a cartoon character like Donald Duck or Mickey Mouse. Sing a children's song that way. Listen to the voices in cartoons to get ideas.

When you are with others, practise speaking like them—in the same register, volume and tempo. Practise meeting others where they are.

Songs for your type

Lullabies, children's songs, folk songs

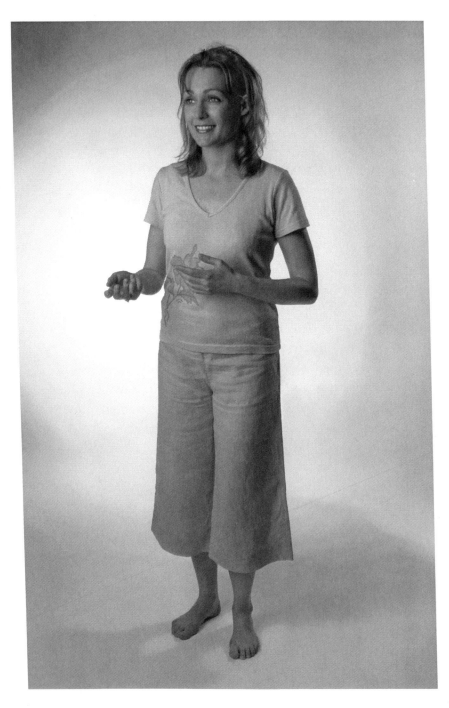

The Cocktail Party Voice

Description

The Cocktail Party Voice speaks in a guarded, calm and super-ficial manner. The voice is usually pitched high or medium-high. Her manner of speaking may strike one as impersonal and prone to cliché. She does not express feelings, but is instead anonymous, hiding behind a façade. For the same reason, the voice is not particularly memorable. The Cocktail Party Voice's problem is that she is so disconnected from her feelings that her life has become barren, and she has difficulty feeling anything at all. We find many of this type among petty office tyrants, stewardesses, and TV and radio personalities.

Explanation

This is quite often a person who has suppressed her deeper feelings so effectively that they can no longer be noticed or even recognised. There is, therefore, a danger of becoming stiff, rigid and numb. There is a great fear of the inner life, which she holds in check by protecting herself with anonymity.

Solution: Predator exercise

Imagine you are a predator—a panther, perhaps. Move across the floor on all fours, paying attention to your body. Begin with an audible, animal breath; then add wild, dangerous and deep growling. Dare to play and to be spontaneous.

Songs for your type

Protest songs, work songs, drinking songs, heroic ballads

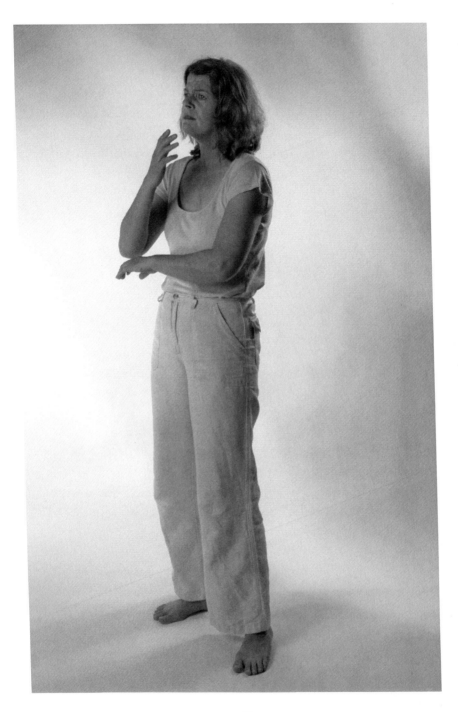

The Hoarse Voice

Description

When there is nothing physiologically wrong with the voice, it is a learned behaviour to be hoarse—that is, something psychic is in play. It is possible to be more or less chronically hoarse; that is, the hoarseness comes and goes. The Hoarse Voice is always identifiable by an airy sound, rough and indistinct. The vocal cords do not close, and air is present in the voice, which makes it disappear or sound smaller.

Explanation

There can be many reasons The Hoarse Voice loses her voice or becomes hoarse. Minor shocks, overexertion and stress can prevent her from expressing her emotions, and that can settle on the voice. If she cannot express herself over a longer period of time, she might experience colds, inflammations or chronic hoarseness. Hoarseness is always a manifestation of feelings that have not been purged and resolved.

Solution: Singing exercise

Start by humming a song you remember from your childhood. Imagine your own voice as a child, before you became hoarse, and see if you can find it again. Then take another song, and sing it like you would for a child. Quietly, calmly and with feeling.

Songs for your type

Religious songs, hymns, songs of praise

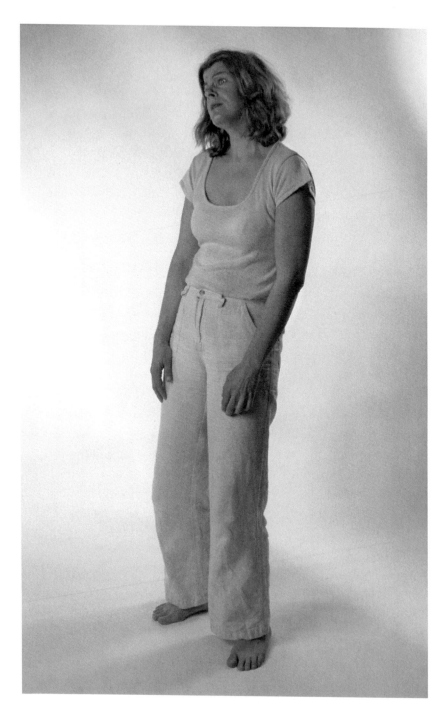

Poor Me

Description

The Poor Me-type often speaks in a high register with a thin voice. His vocal line is descending and slow, with a sighing, whining, complaining or whimpering quality. We recognise this pattern from children who try to get something special from their parents, or who need care and comfort. This type plays at being helpless, and the voice becomes little and pathetic. Even older people can act this part in order to receive things they have become too old and weak to procure themselves.

Explanation

The Poor Me-type is in truth not poor at all, but rather has a great measure of will and power. He uses it, however, to manipulate others. He plays the victim and calls on the whole rescue team available in his world. Here the solution is obviously to stop playing the victim, so he can communicate his needs clearly instead of manipulating others into meeting them.

Solution: Bragging exercise

Pick out some of your virtues and brag about them. Say: I am good. I am good at cooking, reading bedtime stories, etc. Then take a song you know and sing it like a braggart or a world-famous tenor. Exaggerate the effect. If you can do it while others listen, so much the better.

Songs for your type

Erotic songs, songs of praise, heroic odes

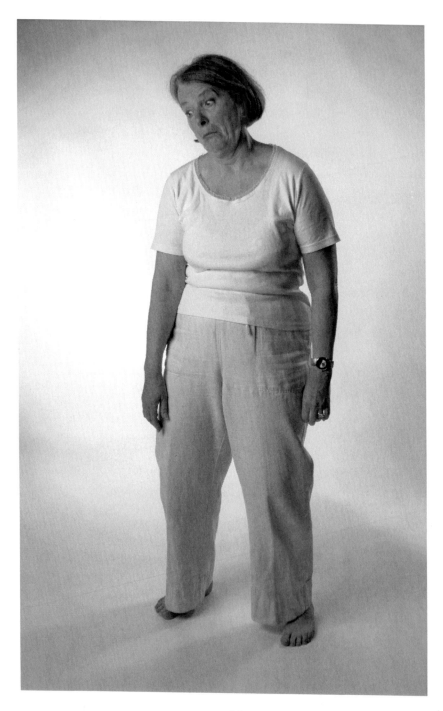

The Killjoy

Description

The Killjoy speaks in a low or middle register, with a tendency to press the voice downward. In the same way, he stifles others, and squeezes the life out of any project. The Killjoy is restrictive and meticulous, and is often found in jobs with great responsibility, in which doing one's duty is highly valued. He can be found in government offices, tax agencies, parking enforcement, etc.

Explanation

The Killjoy is embittered and angry, possibly even hateful. This can result from a failure to acknowledge and address these strong feelings to their real target—for example, a father figure. As a result, this anger and unhappiness seeps out towards everyone around him, causing pain for all involved.

Solution: Champagne exercise

Imagine that your voice is like a champagne bottle being opened. Start with a moderately low note on the vowel [oh], and let your voice glide slowly up, and then release it entirely. You are encouraged to illustrate this movement by using your arms, as though you quickly pulled a sweater over your head and threw it aside. Repeat the exercise many times.

Songs for your type

Songs of joy, sea chanteys, erotic songs

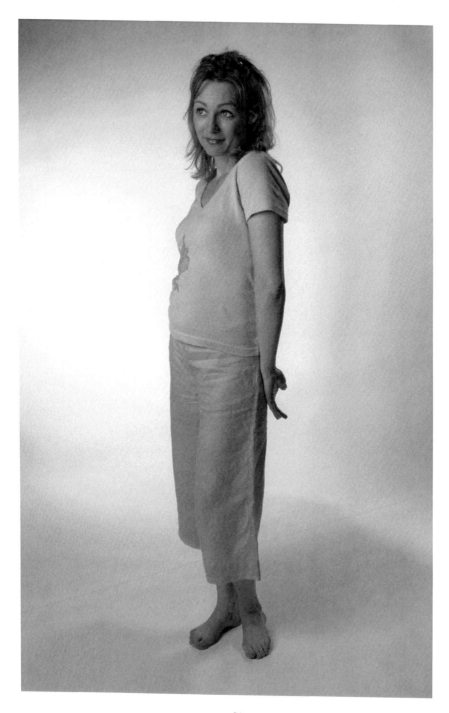

The Beggar

Description

The Beggar speaks with a quiet voice in an average pitch level. She caresses you with her sugary sweet voice, ingratiating and gentle, with a calm tempo and strategically effective pauses. The Beggar manipulates people in her world by giving them what they need. The Beggar, like the Poor Me-type, is a master in making herself irresistible. She makes herself submissive to obtain what she wants, while her counterpart feels like an important benefactor.

Explanation

Those who can perform this unique art have probably learned it out of need. If we cannot get our needs met via direct appeals, we must learn to manipulate. The Beggar has probably been rejected time after time, and therefore has not been able to assert herself. Or, this could have been the usual form of expression in her home growing up, from a submissive mother to a tyrannical father. The Beggar needs to acknowledge her needs and rely on herself to get them met, rather than begging for them.

Solution: Dictator exercise

Practise singing a song or reading a text in a commanding tone of voice. Be direct and demanding, like a dictator or Mother Superior. Sing and speak powerfully. Try this also in a nonsense language.

Songs for your type

Protest songs, working songs, football songs

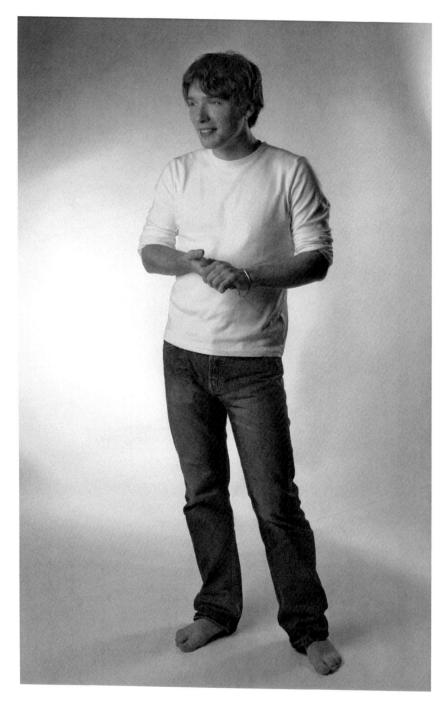

The Seducer

Description

The Seducer is a master in the art of seduction. This type speaks mostly with a low, hushed voice if a man (Jack Nicholson), and with a clear, feline voice if a woman (Marilyn Monroe). Both frequently speak with a slightly husky voice, and in a calm, cunning tempo. This is a voice type that, quite unnoticed, can get right under your skin. Even in extremely dangerous situations, The Seducer can make a personal connection by using his or her uniquely intimate and seemingly trustworthy voice.

Explanation

The Seducer is the subtlest of manipulators. This type appears very self-assured, but can be quite unaware of the methods he uses to seduce others. The Seducer is apt to cross far over another person's boundaries before either party is necessarily aware of it. It strengthens his feeling of identity to have so much power over others. This kind of power or seduction is just one way of receiving acknowledgement from his surroundings, though The Seducer is often unaware of this. He has probably suppressed his own needs, and likely has a low sense of self-worth.

Solution: Cool-off exercise

Take a newspaper and imagine you are reading the day's headlines for the evening news on television. Do it coolly and reservedly, with distance in your voice; then try singing a song with the same kind of anonymity and precision. Practice this every day, and see what it does for you. Practise with others as well, assuming the role of the one who is calm and collected.

Songs for your type

Religious songs, hymns, patriotic songs

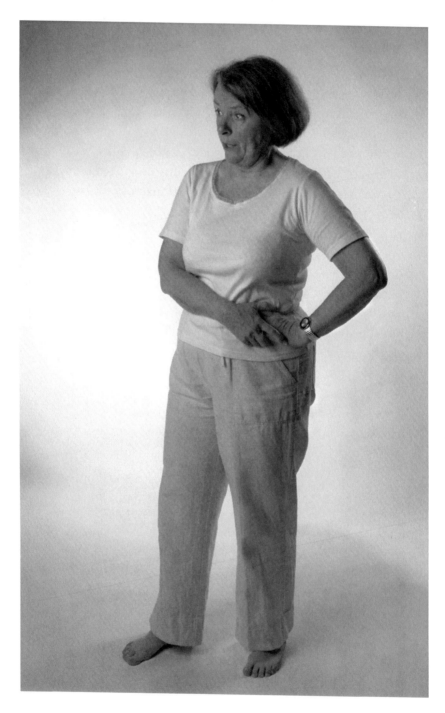

The Throat-Clearer

Description

The Throat-Clearer, as the name suggests, has a bad habit of clearing his throat and coughing discreetly, which can be very irritating to other people. It is often in very specific situations that the need to clear the throat surfaces. Throat-clearing is mostly done unconsciously, and is quite common among many people. It can fatigue and damage the vocal cords.

Explanation

The urge to clear the throat comes from something that is having difficulty coming out. It is a hidden message. Often, The Throat-Clearer has not expressed himself, or has difficulty doing so. Throat-clearing can be accompanied by a great deal of insecurity, repressed anger, petty complaints, irritation and the urge to criticise. As a rule, there is anger over not being heard and taken seriously. Some use throat-clearing to call attention to themselves.

Solution: Sing-your-way-clear exercise

Stand with feet parallel and apart. First, take a few deep breaths and relax. Next, imagine that you need to clear your throat, and notice how that feels. Notice how you contract your stomach and close off the flow of air. Now let some air out in a deep sigh. Do that a few times. Next, sing a song you like and know well, loudly and strongly. Do this many times, especially when you feel the need to clear your throat.

The situation will not always allow you to stand up and sing. In that case, it is better for your voice if you cough properly, than if you clear your throat repeatedly.

Songs for your type

Protest songs, battle songs, heroic odes

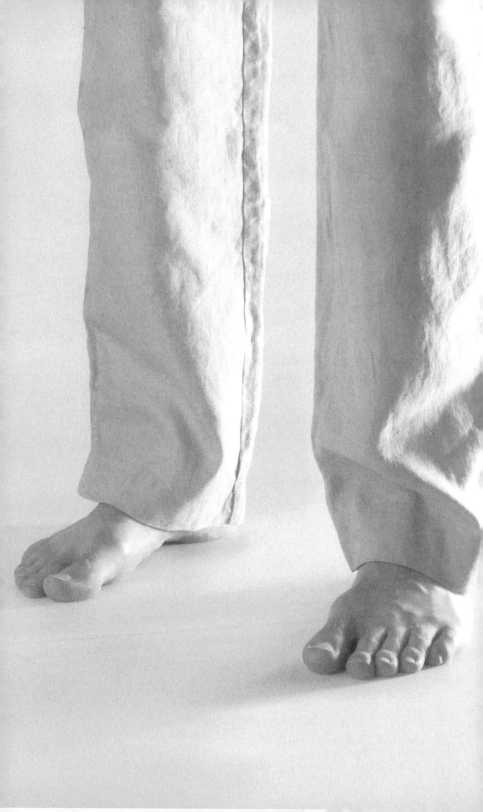

CHAPTER 7

What Will Happen When I Get Started?

How to work with your voice type

1. Sooner or later, most people reach a point where they feel they are stuck in a particular role. Again and again, they find themselves in the same situation with the same type of people— for example, a manipulative female boss. And again and again, they fall into the same role—for example, The Echo, who obligingly allows herself to be manipulated.

2. Figure out which role you play, and really investigate what it leads you to do. Then exaggerate the role. For example, if you tend to have a descending vocal line, exaggerate this, making it even lower, even worse, and observe what happens. These roles are often learned quite early on and operate on a totally unconscious level. That is why it is important to notice what effect they have on you.

3. All roles have a polar opposite. See if you can find yours. If you are a Little Girl, perhaps you should try playing the big bad Wolf. I recommend you first do this as a thought experiment; try and create an internal dialogue between your two opposites. What would they say to each other? Try writing the dialogue down. Next, in safe situations, together with those you know very well, try playing with your opposites. Tell yourself, "Now I'll try playing The Silent Voice." Plan your time, so you don't go overboard at the beginning. Take just five minutes when you are together with others to try playing your role with your new voice. Life is a stage, and we are both actor and director. Allow yourself to use a much greater variety of shades and facets of yourself. This will increase your vitality.

4. As you gain practice with your different voices and different sides of yourself, start switching between them. Work on changing from one role to its polar opposite, also in the company of others. People, and the world around you, will probably react. If you are able, and the situation permits it, exaggerate and play the roles to the hilt. Have fun with them, so they become apparent to those around you. It's possible that you and everyone around you will get a wake up call. You can also choose to explain to your colleagues and friends what you are doing, but there is no guarantee that you will be understood.

5. When you play a role and its opposite, you free up energy to learn something completely new. You liberate new life along with a sudden freedom to choose. In other words, you are no longer bound to your role in the same way as before.

Breaking a habit

Realise that you are about to break a habit that could well be as old as you are; do not be hard on yourself if it does not succeed immediately. Give yourself plenty of time—including time for mistakes—when you are improvising with your voice. It is OK to slip up, just try again. Stop trying to be perfect. Give yourself time to learn and to discover.

On making noise at home

Many people have a hard time giving themselves permission to use their voices fully in their own homes. Noise is taboo—at least, many of the more expressive noises are. We are often so shy about displaying our voices that we do not even allow ourselves to be noisy in our own homes. When we finally do, we may bring our neighbour rushing down, worried that a murder is taking place. The best we can do is to plan our new sound experiments. Put time aside, and inform any neighbours of your intentions. Choose times when you will disturb others as little as possible.

Remember to use your car, the beach or the woods, too—it's magnificent to use your voice surrounded by nature. Try organising sound-hikes in the woods or other trips with others interested in using their voices.

Preconceptions and old ghosts

When we really begin a process of transformation, we are bound to run up against our old preconceptions. Many of us were told we can't carry a tune and were sent to the back of the class with the tone-deaf kids. This is something that has wounded many people so deeply that we never opened our mouths again. When we finally dare to use our voices once more, these unresolved issues return to the surface. Look at the reappearance of all these old ghosts as a chance to resolve them and be free of them. When ghosts come into the light, they lose their power.

Inner resistance

When we seriously desire change and take a step forward in our development, we can also run into our inner resistance. It is as though one part of us wants to believe in life, and the possibilities available to us when we follow our love and inspiration, and the other part won't cooperate at all. Many of us are still influenced by clichés like "no pain, no gain," "life's a bitch," "it's too good to be true," and similar destructive thoughts. We cannot simply eliminate these parts of ourselves. We cannot eliminate our fear of living. We can, however, choose to examine our fear and negative thoughts, accept them, and thereby discover that they usually contain pure life energy. We can also choose to use our inner voice, our intuition and our humour to help us move on.

Support yourself

Have patience with yourself and appreciate yourself. You might say aloud to yourself several times a day, "Isn't it a shame that I was told I couldn't sing? I really deserve now to use my voice to the fullest and get to know it!" Get support from your friends. If you do not have anyone who will support you through this process, find someone who will. The world is full of people. You do not need to spend time with people who do not want what is best for you. Remember to support yourself as well. Join a choir, give a speech, go to drama or voice classes, sing for your partner or your child. Begin where you are and follow your bliss.

Keep on encouraging yourself

When you have worked with your voice for a while, there may come a point when you worry that things cannot keep improving; that your progress is too good to be true. On an unconscious level, we fall back into our old habits, which are familiar and feel safe. The better things are going, the more opposition we unconsciously create inside.

Our unconscious mind tries to create a counterweight. Here is where you will need to make an extra effort. Prepare yourself for these coming setbacks, and continue to encourage yourself as you progress. Affirm and praise yourself.

Rewards of working with your voice

You are now aware of your voice in various situations, and how you use it in relationship to the world around you. In addition, you have been offered exercises and ideas about how you can change your voice: by aligning your comfort zone, strength, vocal line and other elements with your authentic voice. By doing this, you will no longer go along with mind games around you, letting yourself be manipulated. Or perhaps you stop manipulating others. In situations that earlier were difficult to handle, you now are able to adjust so that you exercise free choice instead of engaging in compulsive behaviour. A classic example is the woman whose boss drowns out all his employees (the Trombone-type). He never listens to anyone, steamrolling everyone else. The woman acquires a vanishing Little Girl voice in this situation, and then she is silenced entirely. After appropriate voice work she is now able to stick to her guns and use her voice in her proper comfort zone—deeper and more adult—and can assert herself and not let herself be bullied.

Another example is the self-sacrificing man married to a Poor-Me type. She sighs and complains in a squeaky voice, and he answers with the controlled and pressured voice of one with a great burden of responsibility. His voice work will revolve around giving up responsibility for his wife's issues, releasing his voice and the pressure on it, so that it becomes lighter and freer. This also prompts her to take responsibility for herself. Her voice will become darker and more powerful.

Still, it is not always the case that our surroundings desire the same change and development that we do. You should be prepared for the possibility that your new voice—your new style—will not be met with universal applause. So prepare yourself for the reaction from your environment.

Take your time

It is important that you realise that it takes time to get results. Look at the work as a worthwhile process you are going through. The voice you have imposed on yourself is, as a rule, one that was learned through many years of training, and will require time to be superseded by a new and better one. Have faith in the process, and most importantly, be kind to yourself.

It is also essential that you do not move too fast. In the worst case, you risk losing some relationships that are important to you, or that you cannot afford to lose. For example, you might risk being fired if you bravely instigate a confrontational voice-duel with your boss. So be attentive. Weigh each situation carefully before attempting challenging voice changes, and be sure you are ready to accept the consequences that may result.

Listen to other voices, too

Try to sharpen your awareness of other people's voices. What do they do with their voices that provokes a reaction in you? How do you let yourself be influenced? Perhaps you meet a Wolf voice, which causes you to lose track of the important ideas and arguments you had prepared. Or does a Waterfall drown you out, right when you have something vital to say? Just as your work with your own voice is important, so is attentiveness to how others' voices affect you.

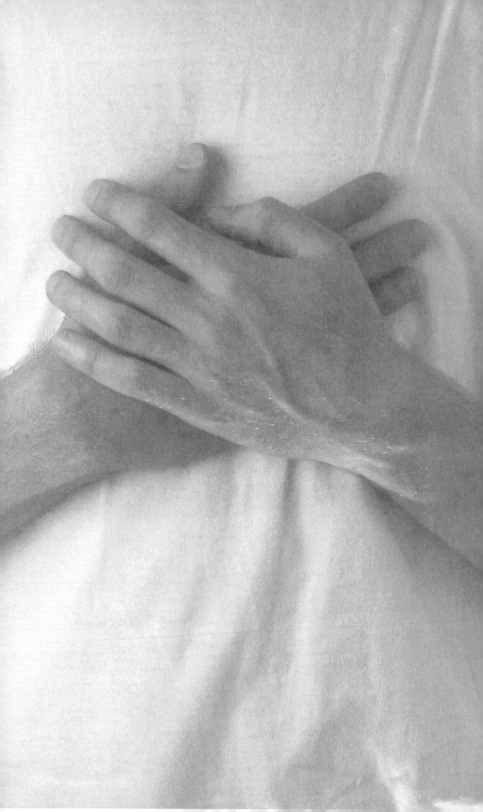

CHAPTER 8

The Voice and the Universe

Voice, dialect and identity

Through all ages, human beings have formed social, cultural and geographic groups. The globe is divided into countries with precise boundaries, which are divided again into cities, boroughs, neighbourhoods and streets where families live, like a series of Chinese boxes. Within each family, distinctive traditions are learned and inherited, which make up the family's "blueprint." This encompasses the sound of the voice, the dialect and a unique way of talking to and with each other.

Every country has its own language, understood by the country's inhabitants, but—historically, anyway—not by those from outside. Language is the psychic borderline, territory and ecosystem. With our language we define the group of individuals to which we belong. We live here, we sound like this, we look like this, we do this, we don't do that. Within one country we have regions with their own dialect, their own language: think of the differences between a gentleman from Surrey, a coal miner from the North, and a Cockney girl from London. Language reveals your geographical location and your surroundings, that is to say, your roots. Language will also tell us about your status and rank—if you grew up on an earl's estate or on a housing estate, in Chelsea or Hackney. The sum of all this contributes to defining our roles and identity.

Language, dialect and jargon can be analysed in these ways: which "melody" is sung here? What does it reveal? Each time we as individuals enter into a new community, we must decide either to sing in harmony with that community, or strike our own unique note—knowing that the latter choice may cause problems, or even necessitate our withdrawal from that community. But there is also a third possibility: we can influence the sound picture, and change the key, as it were.

Within the family unit it is natural that children speak like their parents. But not only are language, dialect, particular forms and figures of speech learned from mother and father, but also register, inflection, volume and etiquette.

How many times have we heard, when a stranger phones, something like: "My goodness, I thought you were your father—you sound almost identical!" Even when we take short or long trips away from home, we are influenced by the vocal sound and particular traditions of the locals—for example, the daughter who comes home from summer vacation and maintains a "foreign" accent and slang for a week or so afterwards.

Every time we enter a group, we adapt to the tone being struck: the presiding norm. Sometimes we are comfortable with this "tone" and sometimes we must leave the group and find a new one that does more to strengthen our identity.

Voices of those we love and hate

There is a natural explanation for everything—even the simple fact that each of us is wild about some people and some voices, and cannot stand others.

This has a lot to do with projection. That is, we often are attracted and repelled by persons who represent sides of ourselves that we either are not conscious of, or do not express. They can be admirable qualities we do not yet know we possess, or unpleasant qualities that we are unaware of and therefore greatly irritate us when we encounter them in others.

When we are attracted by The Trombone-type, for example, it is not because we literally feel a need to go around and overwhelm everyone else; but perhaps we do need to improve our ability to have an impact, and know this subconsciously. In other words, we are attracted and stimulated by qualities we perhaps possess, but are not yet living out.

Think of a well-known person you either adore or cannot abide. When we experience strong antipathy or sympathy, it is often prompted by parts of ourselves we have not yet faced up to. The good thing about projection is that we can catch a glimpse of sides of ourselves we didn't know we had, and can become fuller human beings by claiming them for ourselves. This can be put more philosophically by saying that human development is based upon the recreation of a lost whole, which we all unconsciously remember and long for; and which also causes men and women to be stubbornly attracted to each other. That lost whole, which persistently causes opposites to attract.

When the artist feels what you should feel

There is also a large measure of projection in the relationship between artist and audience. Some people still believe that you need to be a professional in order to take voice lessons. There seems to be a broad consensus that you have to be good first. And if you are not good, then you should instead go and listen to the people who are. This is how we can get trapped in the audience role. We project all our unfulfilled longings and dreams on the performers. But we limit ourselves in this way, which may mean we never deploy our own valuable, creative powers.

On the other hand, it is the artist's privilege to test her own boundaries. She can live out all her foul feelings, and indulge her need for bizarre behaviour, wildness and childishness. Behaviour that in the real world would be taboo is permitted and even rewarded here. But that does not mean that artists are necessarily whole and balanced human beings. In the world of the arts, it is easy to find people who are stuck in certain roles. You can find the rock singer with a tight, closed and restricted sound—in other words, with tension in the root of the tongue. Precisely this type of singing is legitimised because it suits the style, but it can cause a singer to stay permanently out of balance. You can find an opera singer with beautiful raw vocal material, but who traps himself in a Trombone-type, drowning out all others. He measures his worth in volume, and all other details and nuances are lost.

If we look at ourselves and at our fellow human beings through this lens, we will discover that it is an error and an illusion to believe that we can be divided as enemies and opponents.

We are in essence connected, because we are all comprised of both good and evil. We are comprised of all sides, which are hidden in shadows; it is only when we realise that the fundamental conflict is primarily within ourselves that we can accommodate other human beings. We will be in a position to ascend to a higher plane, where we will be free individuals and at the same time deeply interconnected.

It is on this plane that the human voice—its sound—is capable of unifying people across cultures, languages and social backgrounds.

The voice through time

Time plays a critical role when we speak of the voice. Think of your voice as a child as compared to your voice as an adult. Or look at any human's life cycle—childhood, youth, adulthood, old age—and see how the voice changes with time, with age. Some people's voices are unrecognisable when they get older, while others seem not to have changed much at all. There can be individual differences, but whether great or small, change does occur.

Different time periods have also affected the human voice. Going back to the Stone Age, we can presume the survival instinct was dominant. Hunting and reproduction would have played the largest roles. So what did Stone Age humans use their voices for? What was their communication based on, and what was it like?

It is probable that the voice was used more primitively: in a more authentic way, perhaps, employing unarticulated sounds to accompany hunting, food or mating. The inner human—this "natural man"—no doubt lived more fully through instincts and senses than modern humans, who have learned language and structure. In other words, back then we were more body than mind, more nature than culture.

Going forward a bit in history, it would be exciting to know how the Vikings sounded. We would know today, if back then it had been possible to make recordings, but instead we can only imagine. From their body types we could guess some general characteristics: powerful, direct, with deep voices, especially among the men. They were known for their courage (at least the large numbers who journeyed out to conquer other lands were); this trait might indicate a strong forward motion in their speech.

The Victorian era is another exciting time to imagine the interactions between society's norms and people's voices. Did the many controls, taboos and repressed emotions influence how people spoke? And if so, how? Again, we can only speculate.

We can follow language much farther back than we can follow vocal sound. The old papyrus scrolls can be dated to nearly 4000 years ago, but human voice use can only be traced back to the invention of recording technology.

In the first "talkie" films we can hear voices trying to sound correct, respectable and educated. The voices display a slow, clear articulation in a comfortable, middle register; no extreme expression of emotion or dynamics; and clear boundaries. This is a reflection of the era's respectable bourgeoisie; depicting the lower classes was still considered taboo. Today, we show a much broader view of society. Both radio and TV carry a wide variety of language usage, jargon and dialects. The tempo of the voice is much faster, reflecting the more stressed and pressured lifestyle of our time. Fortunately, however, our tolerance of a freer use of the voice has also increased.

New gender roles—new voices

Most people react instinctively to high voices as "feminine" and deep voices as "masculine." This obviously does not mean that women cannot have deep voices or men cannot have high voices. In my experience and in my work with the voice, however, I have found that our associations on this point are unambiguous. It is an inheritance we carry with us. Just as girls play with dolls and boys with trucks, no matter how their parents try to influence them otherwise: it is archetypal.

In fact, in our culture, we have reshuffled our ideals and expectations of how men and women should sound for generations. And we still do. Since it has become permissible for women to integrate more of the masculine in their personalities— becoming more varied and nuanced—women's voices have displayed more strength and power, using the deeper and rawer registers that formerly were reserved for men. Take for example a woman, who after a course in voice study really had accessed the raw strength of her voice. She says, "Late one night, when I was on my way home from a party, I was followed by a man. He came closer and closer to me, until I could nearly smell his sweat. Determined, I turned around and screamed at him for all I was worth. He must have gotten a fright, because he took off." The woman in question is petite and thin (but with strong vocal cords), and it obviously came as a surprise to that man that she could possess that kind of power.

In the same way, as men dare to integrate a feminine side into their personalities, they gain more access to the higher, sensitive and softer qualities of their voices. Of course, this does not make them less masculine.

A varied view of gender roles simply helps us to dare to make use of more sides of our voices. In other words, we gain access to greater nuance.

The balance between female and male voices

When we change our voices, as in the example of the woman who gained more raw strength and depth in her voice, we automatically influence the opposite sex. In interactions with another person, we are attracted to (as described earlier) an opposite pole; for example, an old-fashioned male chauvinist needs a submissive woman. A coy, girlish voice calls out for a big bad wolf. If we are able to change these roles by changing our voices, a new balance will be struck between the sexes. A resonant, centred voice in its natural register influences its environment much more than we think. It will no longer be possible for the other party to persist in a manipulative role-play. You will get the answers you seek. When you change your voice, you change your personality, and thereby provoke change in your surroundings.

The voice of the future: weapon or cure?

We live in an era that confronts us with monumental change in many important areas. We, along with our Earth, are facing ecological and psychic crises. Technology increasingly supplants human work in ways amounting to a paradigm shift. The old world, a world oriented toward outward concerns like status, money, material possessions, fame, work, food, etc., is about to disappear. We are turning our eyes toward a new world and new societal values, oriented toward inner human resources, with greater emphasis on the feminine and the universal.

These new global impulses will also have an impact on the voice. Hopefully, there will be more research into the magic of voice and sound, and the myriad ways we can use them. Here I am referring especially to the voice as a tool for healing. Specific sound frequencies can affect particular bodily organs. Already, there are vocal sounds for calming, sounds for awakening, sounds that can eliminate plantar warts and headaches, and sounds that can cause change on a cellular level. It is clear that with the right research we will be able to heal even serious illnesses. But no one can know exactly how the voice will be used in the future—we can only guess.

David Lynch, in the science fiction film *Dune,* offers an exciting vision of what the voice might be used for. The main character, a super-creature and new Messiah, has parapsychological abilities, including a voice with hypnotic power. He uses it as a weapon, illustrated in the film with an unusually low register. We hear in the film, "Some thoughts have a certain sound, thought being equivalent to a form... Through sound and motion, you will be able to paralyse nerves, shatter bones, set fires...." This is obviously an action film with many violent scenes, where the voice is used as a weapon to battle the enemy (in service of a good cause, of course), but the perspective is nevertheless exciting. If in the future we can influence matter with sound, it will have wide-ranging consequences. Think of what it might mean in the health sector. Imagine using sound as a tool for surgery: sound-surgery!

Or perhaps we will discover sound frequencies that influence the atmosphere, so that we could protect ourselves from polluted air or harmful radiation. It would require exhaustive research to determine which sound frequencies could match corresponding vibrations in—for example—a cancerous tumour. It would also demand a change of awareness and great human responsibility to administer such a powerful tool. These ideas belong to the future; and yet this future is being prepared already, right now.

CHAPTER 9

Cases

These cases are examples. For example, just because you have a Wolf-type voice, it does not necessarily follow that you have the same background or psychological traits as those described here. There are many possible variations within the same voice type.

The Trombone

Jim had studied voice with some of the top singing teachers at home and abroad. He had made a name for himself in musicals and was getting more and more jobs in both straight and musical theatre. Jim's full-bodied bass-baritone boomed when he started a tone way down in his gluteus muscles. He loved to stand stark naked in front of the mirror, to "feel my life energy and sing through my body," as he said. He called it "channel-singing," with a goofy smile. He felt a joyful and euphoric sensation when his body became a channel for something large and spiritual.

Jim had a tendency to exaggerate almost everything he did, the better to be aware of his body—or, more probably, the better to *avoid* being aware of his body. It was always Jim you heard first at a party, and Jim who was the last to leave—he might even do the dishes when everyone else had gone home.

Jim endured, and Jim persevered. He filled in the empty spaces. He was tenacious.

Deep down, he knew that he was afraid: afraid of the ordinary, afraid of not being good enough, afraid of hurting others and, most of all, afraid of being hurt himself. He was afraid of being a burden and being wrong and being stupid. The last was the worst. In fact, he got angry just thinking about it: angry with himself for feeling stupid and afraid. He had to fight his anxiety and man up—puff himself up, in fact—and it could be heard in his voice.

Sometimes he was afraid of arriving late. He developed a habit of coming fifteen to thirty minutes early. He was always on deck, ready and waiting. He was *so* present that he became a caricature, and those around him found him pushy.

Vocal Journey

Jim was a very accomplished singer. Most people found his voice so impressive that they forgot to listen for the finer nuances of the voice. It was not until you were one-on-one with him that you began to discover an entirely different Jim—once, of course, you were able to dissuade him from taking control in his usual way: he was game for anything and everything I suggested; he was eager and enthusiastic; he of course already knew all the exercises we were using, because he had used them in teaching himself, or because he had learned them from this or that famous singing teacher. He was, in the beginning, very busy trying to please me: trying to prove to me (and to himself) that he was good enough.

The voice gave it away.

You could hear it in the way Jim began a tone with that exaggerated energy. It was not an unhealthy, hard glottal attack, which slams the vocal folds together and can cause strain and hoarseness. No—Jim was a trained singer, and his esteemed teachers would have corrected any such tendency long ago. The onset of his voice actually began long before it could be heard. His entire body was in a constant state of readiness for what was to come.

His body was perpetually prepared, sufficiently poised to avert even a nuclear attack.

It was a completely new concept for Jim to create a tone out of nothing (*start-from-zero exercise*), to forget everything he had learned and begin to explore with his voice. It was unsuccessful for a long time, although he continued to come to lessons. At last, it was an emotional cue that allowed him to start his tones in a whole new way. Jim did not expect that anything would come out of his mouth unless he pushed, enlarged and almost violently forced his voice. In the moment when he refrained from pushing, a totally new voice emerged. It trembled; the vocal folds would barely close, and the tone was tiny. Jim broke down in tears. It was that emotion which re-established contact to a very frightened little boy.

Jim's father was strict and authoritarian. He was a deputy judge, and was almost never at home. When he was home, he was preoccupied by his two sons' achievements, especially by the grades they got in school. Jim was a big kid. Even as a little child he was faced with playmates that looked at him disparagingly and teased him for being fat. He frequently started fights with them, which he was able to win because of his strength and size; but he had no real friends at school, and felt very much alone.

His father was both distant and, when he was around, domineering. He had a violent temper, and Jim had on numerous occasions watched his big brother be beaten for failing to live up to their father's expectations.

Jim's father sometimes got a deadly look in his eye, or cleared his throat in a conspicuous way. Jim learned quickly to recognise these warning signs and respond to them by becoming either physically or mentally "invisible."

Through a long process, Jim finally was able to discover a new and different side of his voice.

It demanded his absolute patience, along with understanding and acceptance of his situation. Jim learned how to get in touch with his fragile voice, his angst and his vulnerability, and these now became evident in his voice as *presence*, the ability to produce *nuanced sounds*, and to be able to express feelings of *longing, pain* or *despair*. Combined with Jim's wonderfully trained trombone-like voice, he now had the potential to access a broad palette of expression.

Jim's vocal journey lasted four years, including periods of weekly sessions and periods with no sessions.

Result

Ability to sing quietly and introspectively

Ability to produce nuanced sounds

Better balance between loud and soft tones

Greater emotional expression

The Killjoy

Even though Per tried to sound chipper and happy on his answering machine, as he introduced himself and his fifteen-year-old son Klaus over a background of manly guitar music, his killjoy voice did not abandon him. When you got Per on the phone in person, you could hear how he pressed on his voice, as if to keep all his emotions under tight control. So you knew, at least, what to expect.

You felt a little controlled yourself, talking to him, and you could feel an urge to fight back or defend yourself against something you couldn't quite identify. This feeling lasted long after the call ended.

Sometimes I wondered what would happen if Per stopped pushing his voice down. I had the impression that it might bounce up, and become light like a feather, bright, perhaps even silly and playful.

Per was short and stocky, rather small for a man. He had a good, secure job as a project leader for the municipality. He had a firm handle on most of his life, especially the physical, material side. He was financially secure, with his own house in a posh suburb, a girlfriend he only saw when he wanted to, and a teenage son about to enter a prestigious high school. Per had a good life, and he saw little reason to change it.

But with age he had developed an allergy that affected his bronchi, airways, throat and eyes. At times his eyes could swell up severely, and his voice would sound as if it was smothered in porridge. This really bothered him, because his colleagues at work had begun to notice and even pass remarks about it.

Vocal Journey

When Per contacted me, it was not with a typically direct motivation, but rather with an unconscious seeking. A colleague had heard of my work, and persuaded him to try an approach based on the voice. Per's first voice sessions went by nearly without using the voice for anything but speaking. He categorically avoided singing tones and sounds; every time I suggested an exercise, he interrupted with some idea, and if I tried to make myself heard, he only spoke faster and louder. When I politely confronted him about this phenomenon, it actually stopped, and we were able to work. He did, however, really want to talk about the music he had liked in high school, and about how he had once played guitar in a band.

Per's voice was badly blocked. He had tension in the root of his tongue, meaning the tongue was pulled back in the throat, blocking the flow of air. He also had an "iron torso" around his ribcage. That was how he described it, anyway: a feeling of being imprisoned when he inhaled. We began to investigate this fortress—both prison and protection, of course—with the help of a variety of awareness exercises, breathing techniques and meditative sound exercises in slow motion, which allowed him to feel and sense.

His vulnerability became more and more apparent as he came closer to the grief he had carried around for many years, but had apparently neither acknowledged nor resolved. First, the loss of a playmate he had a close friendship with from 1st to 5th grade, who was killed in a car accident. Then, the loss of a son he had fathered in what he called "a little accident" when he was very young, and had opted to have no contact with. And last but not least, the loss of his wife, whose deep depression caused her to commit suicide.

When Per spoke about these losses, he appeared unmoved; but when he sang or performed sound exercises with his body and his voice, his emotions increasingly broke through, and as they did, he became able to sing both higher and more quietly. It became clear that behind his iron bars and underneath his killjoy personality lay a fine tenor voice.

Per dug out the old 60s songs from his high school days, bought a new guitar and began playing with three others in a band, where they had a great time. Joy has returned to his life through his voice. He has become better at listening, and simply sounds happier. His tendency to push the voice down in order to control his feelings has disappeared, because he is better at allowing them in and expressing them. He now dares to stand by the true register of his voice, namely a lighter, higher one, while also acknowledging his more refined, or feminine, sides.

His allergy has not disappeared, but it has significantly eased.

His vocal journey has so far lasted two years with sessions on average every two weeks.

Result

Obtained access to a higher comfort zone, in the tenor register

Tension in the root of the tongue disappeared

Melody in speaking voice appeared

The Wolf and The Silent Voice

Linda and Henrik had known each other for a year and a half when they decided to move into an apartment together in Copenhagen. Linda, who was five years older than Henrik, was going to business school. She was bright, extroverted and charming. Henrik had not yet decided on a course of study, and had temporarily taken a job in a travel agency. He was tall and dark, with an inscrutable look in his brown eyes. It was as though he had kicked the ball down the field and was waiting for someone else to play on—in other words, for someone else to live his life for him.

And that was exactly what Linda did. She took control of that ball at once and had kept it ever since. She was one who had hit on Henrik; she was the one who suggested they move in together; she was the one who found the apartment, and the one who, with her creativity and good taste, had decorated most of it.

Henrik followed along, silent and consenting. Or was it silent and accusing? With Henrik, one never knew exactly what he was thinking or feeling. At times he created uncomfortable insecurity with his silence, and at other times a stimulating, nearly aphrodisiac, curiosity about himself. Linda felt attracted to the latter. Here, she could use her creativity, her energy—everything she had learned. She buried the uncomfortable insecurity and unconsciously chose not to deal with it.

Henrik profited by this choice. He didn't have to do anything himself. He felt a certain familiar control over the situation, a certain self-satisfaction.

Vocal Journey

Linda's voice was clear, bright and authoritative. It had lots of energy and forward impulse, but also an undertone of anger. She had a wide vocal range, she was musical, and she loved to sing. It was obvious that she had a lot to offer. She was very interested in working with her voice. In the very first sessions she got close to the work that would define this process for her: the theme of power and helplessness.

As a child, Linda had to take responsibility for her mentally fragile mother. Linda was the oldest of three sisters, the one the whole family relied on. She bought the groceries, made dinner, kept house, and took care of her younger siblings. She took on her mother's role, becoming the matriarch, her father's trusted ally: "daddy's big girl," as he called her with pride. She received her father's positive attention and recognition in the role of an adult woman. She developed qualities like creativity, decisiveness and responsibility, qualities which were audible in her "Wolf" voice—even if they are positive.

Linda had power and drive in her voice, but had a harder time singing quietly and otherwise producing tones with just the very edges of the vocal cords. Her voice was also slightly rigid or stiff, lacking flexibility and mobility. It was easy for Linda to take responsibility and leadership; but could she also give them away?

Or even set them aside? It was little wounded Linda, who always had to take responsibility for everyone else, but who in reality never had the opportunity to feel helpless. That should have been natural for a girl in her situation, who lacked the care of her mother and the feeling of an adult taking full responsibility for her. Unconsciously, she longed to be on the receiving end of things, and the sound lay hidden in these emotions.

We worked with the *release-the-tone exercise*, the *seize-the-energy exercise*, the *stop-the-energy exercise* and the *onset exercise* so that Linda could acquire a new balance between power and helplessness, giving and receiving.

Linda's voice, once bright and authoritative, became capable of softness, intimacy and sensuality, too. She acquired additional nuances in her voices when she surrendered her power. Linda was especially able to soften her voice when singing, lending greater emotional power to expressions of loss, longing or closeness. The most beautiful expression of wholeness was achieved when she improvised in the *follow-the-energy exercise.*

The vocal journey lasted six months with sessions every three weeks.

Result

Greater flexibility and mobility in the voice
Better balance between loud and soft tones
Ability to sing with intimacy and sensuality in the voice

The Silent Voice

Henrik's voice sounded brittle, airy and boyishly changeable, with pauses that seemed to signal a hesitant attitude as well as a kind of dismissiveness. He never spoke much, was often silent and rarely got worked up. It was a pleasant voice, since he never spoke too loudly, but at the same time a listener felt oddly paralysed, as though his hesitant silence was contagious. On the other hand, when once in a great while he did get upset, it came in dramatic explosions that shook those around him.

But that was rare. Mostly, Henrik's anger was expressed in indirect ways.

He could punish others with the silent treatment or freeze them out entirely; even better, he could get them to do things for him, allowing them to think they were the cause of his anger.

Vocal Journey

Henrik's voice was filled with a repressed or understated rage that was as unacknowledged as his need for control and power.

He needed to be convinced to get in the game and get a hold of the power of his voice; this was difficult, since he had created a pattern of silence and defiant anger. First, to ask him to give voice to his anger was to ask him to expose his inmost self; and that there should also be witnesses to this pushed his boundaries intolerably. These two conditions proved to be a critical turning point for Henrik.

Henrik began with the *Samurai exercise*—first with words, which are more concrete than sound alone. Sound can seem more "dangerous" because it is pure energy, with direct access to the body and to the emotions.

The words and pictures that came to the surface surprised Henrik with how raw and primitive they were. After a while, Henrik began to release a riot of nonverbal sounds, accompanied by the feelings of anger—but also of humour and joy—that were trapped in his body.

Henrik's new access to his anger could be heard in the greater impact and strength his voice now possessed; it also meant that his articulation got significantly better. Consonants especially became clearer in his spoken voice. Consonants define rhythm in speech, while vowels create the melody. Vowels carry content, flowing and boundless, while consonants form the boundaries and structure.

Henrik's parents divorced when he was eight years old at his father's request. He had lived a double life with other women and left Henrik's mother with three children.

Henrik described his father as a man of few words who had little contact with his feelings, and had difficulty expressing himself. Henrik remembered the atmosphere as a child sitting at the dinner table: an icy silence reigned between his parents. Later, there was silence around the divorce, and silence again when Henrik's father became seriously ill and died at the age of 64. This was not a family that spoke to each other.

When Henrik broke his own pattern of silence, it allowed playfulness, creativity and humour to crop up in his voice.

Henrik, who had never used his voice for anything except keeping silent and holding back, now had the urge to sing. He started with simple children's songs he remembered from school days, but later tried many different genres, including rock, classical, standards and jazz. It was quite contrary to their usual roles when Henrik, not Linda, took the initiative to suggest they sing together.

This vocal journey lasted two years with sessions once a month.

Result

Greater power and volume
Better articulation
Begins to sing

The Wolf Meets The Silent Voice

Linda and Henrik's relationship pushed each of them to the extremes of their learned tendencies; they influenced each other such that their roles became amplified or worsened. The more resourceful and decisive Linda was, the more silent and withdrawn Henrik became, and vice versa. Outwardly, it was Linda who had the power and the energy, with her headlong, aggressive vocal power, and Henrik who was passive and helpless, with his withheld, weak and silent voice. On the unconscious, hidden level, it was exactly the opposite.

Linda dared not feel and acknowledge her helplessness; Henrik dared not feel and acknowledge his power and desire for control.

When they began to sing together, they found a common platform, a kind of playground. This freed them from their fixed roles and allowed them to experiment and find new vocal expressions—new roles. It was in this nonverbal space, a vocal space, that they could escape all their clichés and behavioural patterns.

Linda and Henrik came to sessions together for nine months, once every three weeks.

The Waterfall

The sound of Irene's harried stiletto heels reached my ear before the doorbell did. And even before I opened it, I could hear her bright and slightly shrill voice talking energetically. I wondered whether she had bumped into the mailman or asked the neighbour for directions. I opened the door, and, still speaking into her cell phone, Irene smiled and nodded to me as she walked into the apartment. She dug feverishly in her purse, turned off the cell, turned it on again, turned it off again, and checked her face in the mirror, all without interrupting a long string of—mostly incomplete—sentences. She gasped for air, her voice cracked, and she suddenly fell silent. "Sorry about that," she said. "I should have left the office earlier." She had arrived 20 minutes late for her first voice session, to which her boss had referred her. Irene was a secretary in a large computer company. She had difficulty being listened to and taken seriously. Her boss, a man much younger than herself, expressed it a bit differently. He thought she could stand to sound a bit more "bitchy," with more punch in her voice, so that clients could sense that she had authority.

In reality, though, her endless jabbering often irritated him. She spoke like a waterfall, he thought, and no one wanted to listen to her. On the other hand, she was very competent in written tasks, and he did not want to lose her perceptive and professional understanding of the field. For this reason he had earlier sent her on a course in personal effectiveness, but it did not seem to have had much effect besides helping her find a new boyfriend, with whom she was very preoccupied.

Vocal Journey

Irene's voice was as frenzied as she was. Her breath was much too high in her body, and did not extend down to her diaphragm or abdominal muscles. Her body was tense, especially her neck and throat muscles. These are the same symptoms we expect to see in persons under a lot of pressure or stress: the breath creeps higher and higher in the body, while muscle tension increases, especially in the neck and throat. There is also a direct parallel to the physical reactions experienced during anxiety or emotional shock, but to a lesser degree.

Irene's voice was obviously affected by her shallow, short breaths. She did not take in enough air in her inhalation; it was almost absent, and left her gasping for breath.

Her range also shifted higher, with increasing shrillness; she had no power or authority in her voice; and her sound quality was flat, lacking fullness and tending to crack.

Irene's voice changed noticeably the moment she used it to

sing. Here she was forced to breathe fully when challenged for example to sing a long, low note on "ah" in the *follow-through exercise*. The next inhalation was almost automatically deep and sustained, which was exactly what she needed. She became more mentally present and calmed down, which enabled her to get in better touch with her body. Before this, there was a cloud of unrest and confusion around her, which had obscured who she really was.

After this we were able to work towards getting her breathing deep into the body, in contact with the vital power we are all born with. We did this with the help of the *own-your-space exercise*, the *boundary exercise*, the *say-no exercise*, and the *hold-your-ground song*.

Irene's voice underwent a marked change. It fell into place in a lower comfort zone, a slower tempo, and a fuller and warmer sound. She is still working on it, so it is too early to draw conclusions; but she has broken free of her hectic nature and her habit of speaking like a waterfall. She appears much calmer and more attentive. Although she once in a while falls into her old chaotic habits, she is also able to stop herself, take a deep breath, and make a different choice.

This vocal journey has lasted nine months and continues with regular sessions every three weeks.

The Brake

The first time Anna contacted me, she told me over the phone that she was very tense in her throat and neck. I noticed that she had a very deep voice, as well as a tendency to slow down or stop when speaking, as though she expected to be interrupted. I also noticed that her voice sometimes changed entirely, becoming bright, vulnerable and small; I thought these were valuable qualities that ought to be respected. She signed up for an introductory workshop, and following that participated in both long-term group and individual work.

An important look back

One of Anna's earliest memories of her voice came back to her as she was on her way to our first class meeting. One of the day's agenda points was that participants should share a bit about their relationship to their own voice. This triggered childhood memories of how she had a lower voice than most girls, and was often taken for a man, especially on the telephone.

When Anna was about eight years old, her class was going to record a story on tape to be sent to children in another school. She was given the role of narrator, and another girl had the role of "the bear." When the tape was played back, it sounded ridiculous: the bear spoke with a very bright girl's voice, while the narrator growled like a bear. But no one said anything.

Anna told me that she felt uncomfortable and worried that she was not normal, a feeling that had returned many times since in her life. Earlier she had been able to laugh it off, but now was more and more likely to get angry. In other words, she had started to react, which was both reasonable and understandable.

Little Anna

Anna had learned a very masculine behavioural pattern, and spoke almost like a man. In many of our exercises she was confronted with her determination and tendency to push herself hard. At the same time she had difficulty producing childlike sounds, like whimpering or baby talk. While she had a hard time getting in touch with the little girl in her, she had a deep need to do so. She had to process a lot of negative thoughts about herself before she really dared to express these sounds. When she finally had a breakthrough with her sound, it was both powerful and intense, and allowed her to gain greater insight.

The way home

Anna said that when she left voice class, she was often full of self-confidence, strength and energy; but after a little while the euphoria dissipated and made room for deeper emotions.

She described it as a depression creeping in. Her body got heavier and heavier, and a grey, unbearable heaviness spread out from her heart, ending in tears.

She was mourning for her womanhood: despite her 34 years, she had had no sense of being a woman. For Anna, having a woman's body had been associated with a strong feeling of shame.

At that moment Anna discovered that she was starting from scratch. She began to ask her friends what they thought womanhood was and is. It took a while before she realised that she could not really use their answers, but had to find her own way to her own womanhood.

Some negative thoughts—the inner judge
My concentration fails.

I'm not in touch with myself.

Everyone else has a better, more enjoyable voice than I do.

I don't understand the instructions.

It makes me uncomfortable that others hear my voice in voice class.

When I am myself, I am domineering and "too much" for the others.

New, positive self-affirmations
This is how I feel, and this is how I sound.

I dare to be fully myself.

I dare to use my voice and be heard by others.

I dare to say no and to use the power of my voice.

I feel sure of myself, sure of my voice.

Comments
Anna speaks with a dark, low voice and often holds back with her sound in vocal exercises, in the same way she holds her voice

back, and holds her voice down.

Her body language is characterised by arms stuck in close to the body; she keeps to the edges of a group, along the walls, trying to make herself invisible. It is my impression that Anna does not feel at home in her vocal comfort zone—that she was not born with a dark voice. She has made her voice dark, and surely had her reasons for doing so. A lighter voice would probably have been undervalued or even rejected in her family. To survive, it was therefore necessary to repress an entire part of her voice, corresponding to an entire part of herself and her identity.

It is in this area that I see her potential developmental work: to get acquainted with her higher register, her lighter voice, and to explore all of its possibilities and attributes as though it were a part of her own hidden personality and hidden womanhood. She must go all the way back to the time when she repressed her light voice. The little girl and the big girl correspond to the little voice and the big voice: they must be found. These qualities and the renewed life that comes with them must be brought forward into the present.

Anna also needs to dare to give up her martyr role and thereby her pressure on herself. She says, for example, "I use up loads of energy trying to be myself in the present, trying to avoid pushing myself all the time to achieve something." Physically, Anna is aware of a feeling of being tight and tense in her chest, as well as of a new sensation in her left arm. She says, "I need to work with my arms and my sound, my roar and my laughter!" In other words, she needs to free up her arms and chest, to stand tall and accept more attention for being the woman and the human being she is, along with her whole self and her whole sound.

Result

Releases control
Obtains access to her high, light voice and dares to use it
Released flow of speech without braking

The Beggar

Andreas arrived in my group with a great need to express himself. As I got to know him, it was not hard to see why. He had been an incredibly affectionate child, but his mother was unable to accommodate his love, and rejected him again and again. As a result, he began to both stammer and squint at the age of three. In this way, he shouldered the guilt for his mother's rejection. There had to be something wrong with *him*, so he created reasons not to be seen (the squint) or heard (the stammer). This handicap provided further proof that there really was something wrong with him.

Paradoxically, he now discovered that this led to increased attention from his mother, since she was now obliged to deal with the problem by taking him to specialists such as speech therapists. Andreas says, "It was apparently easier for my mother to relate to a 'problem' child than a healthy one." He adopted this habit, this contrary way of getting love and acceptance from his mother, and thereby laid the foundation for the way he would live his life.

Mixed messages

Andreas learned the following negative behaviour: "When I express myself, I will be rejected; so I must deny myself by becoming difficult and wrong. In this way, I will receive love and acceptance." Later, this theme revealed itself in group sessions. Every time Andreas wanted to open up and express himself as he was, with all the emotions he possessed, using the life and power of his voice, he experienced fear of rejection. Every time he approached his authentic form of expression, the anxiety arose: "If I showed how I really am, people would distance themselves!" It is clear that the voice, which was of course his wounded means of expression, was a door to real growth. The more sound he got out, the better he felt.

A boundary is broken down

In an exercise where the arms are lifted up over the head, completely innocently, Andreas felt his boundaries being stretched. His arms stiffened at the horizontal, and did not want to go any higher. He did finish the movement, however, and experienced a catharsis. The gesture reminded him of a child reaching out for his mother. Physically, he had not been able to do this exercise for a long time.

Untapped sound

Andreas says, "As a child I loved to play with a particular sound, that real Tarzan-sound."

I perceived Andreas to be a very resourceful person, who had a great deal to share. When his fierce anger was permitted, it was like a tornado of sound that filled the room; when his more sensitive side was expressed in a quiet, intense sound, there was no doubt he was a musician. It was this sound, untapped for many years, which now surfaced with an enormous power.

Rapprochement

Again and again in his life, Andreas knew the feeling of needing to beg his way to acceptance. In many relationships, the problem was needing to prove he was "good enough," or feeling like he needed to disprove something else. The theme of rejection was especially prominent in his relationships with women: he won their love by rejecting them and appearing disinterested. Of course, these were women who themselves had a problem with this kind of pattern.

Gradually, as he was able to integrate more and more of his vocal resources and be heard by others in the group, Andreas achieved greater self-acceptance, and thereby a new sense of freedom. This resulted in some new encounters with women in which, instead of trying to win their love and acceptance through a negative pattern, as in the past, he dared to come right out and tell them of his joy and love. He described it beautifully himself: "As love arrives, condemnation disappears." So by exploring the unexpressed, hidden sides of the voice—his laughter, growling, shouts of joy and singing—Andreas took a step closer to his authentic life, along with the love and closeness that he and all of us long for.

Result

Greater vocal volume and power
Larger vocal range (more notes)
Quicker tempo
More nuances in the voice

Bibliography

Eugenio Barba, *Beyond the Floating Islands*

Barbara Ann Brennon, *Hands of Light*

Barbara Ann Brennon, *Light Emerging*

Christine Byriel and Sten Byriel, *Se mig! - hør mig!*

Don Campbell, *The Mozart Effect*

Melba Colgrove, Harold H. Bloomfield and Peter McWilliams, *How to Survive the Loss of a Love*

Alv A. Dahl and Aud Dalsegg, *Charmer and Tyrant*

Githa Ben David, *Tonen fra Himlen*

Marianne Davidsen-Nielsen and Nini Leick, *Healing Pain: Attachment, Loss and Grief Therapy*

Olivea Dewhurst-Maddock, *The Book of Sound Therapy*

Karlfried Graf von Dürckheim, *Hara: The Vital Center of Man*

Shakti Gawain, *The Path of Transformation*

Theo Gimbel, *Healing Through Colour*

Edward T. Hall, *The Silent Language, The Hidden Dimension*

Peter Michael Hamel, *Through Music to the Self*

Jan Johansen and Niels Toft, *Sig hvad du mener*

Peter Levine, *Waking the Tiger: Healing Trauma*

Asger Lorentsen, *Hjertets healende lys*

Anna and Alexander Mauthner, *Conversations with Bob Moore*

Alice Miller, *Thou Shalt Not Be Aware*

Alice Miller, *For Your Own Good: Hidden Cruelty in Child-rearing and the Roots of Violence*

Alice Miller, *Banished Knowledge*

Bent Ølgaard, *Kommunikation og økomentale systemer, ifølge Gregory Bateson*

Marshall B. Rosenberg, *Nonviolent Communication: A Language of Life*

Dane Rudhyar, *The Magic of Tone and the Art of Music*

Anette Tholstrup, *Det lille barn og dig*

Eskild Tjalve, Marianne Suhr and Gurli Ohm Hernø, *Forvandling*

Eckhart Tolle, *The Power of Now: A Guide to Spiritual Enlightenment*

AYNI
BOOKS

"Ayni" is a Quechua word meaning "reciprocity" – sharing, giving and receiving – whatever you give out comes back to you. To be in Ayni is to be in balance, harmony and right relationship with oneself and nature, of which we are all an intrinsic part. Complementary and Alternative approaches to health and well-being essentially follow a holistic model, within which one is given support and encouragement to move towards a state of balance, true health and wholeness, ultimately leading to the awareness of one's unique place in the Universal jigsaw of life – Ayni, in fact.